10,000 Ad

Louis Cataldie, MD

Dedicated to

Christopher L. Cataldie, RN
*My son who has chosen to dedicate his life to the
healing art and science of medicine.*

And to

Joseph R. Cataldie, JD
*My son who has chosen to dedicate his life to family
and healthcare law.*

Biographical Sketch

Louis Cataldie, MD

Dr. Louis Cataldie, a native of Louisiana, received his Medical Degree from LSU Medical School in New Orleans. He has extensive clinical and administrative experience in Addiction Medicine and is a Diplomate of the American Board of Addiction Medicine. He has been in the field of addiction medicine for over thirty years. His first encounter with the recovery process began on June 28, 1978. Dr. Cataldie has developed and served as Medical Director of several successful recovery programs for both adults and adolescents. He was a consultant to the White House on adolescent inhalant abuse during the Reagan years.

Dr. Cataldie previously served as Medical Director for the Office of Addictive Disorders for the State of Louisiana. He is a published author and is long recognized as an expert in the field of addiction medicine. Dr. Cataldie is also a sought-after pubic speaker on the diseases of addiction.

In 2005, he was appointed Medical Examiner for the State of Louisiana and the Incident Commander of the Family Assistance Center for Hurricane Katrina. He was in charge of the recovery and identification of deceased victims of Katrina and for locating over 26,000 missing/displaced persons. Upon completion of that mission, he returned to the field of Addiction Medicine.

He is actively involved in community service and serves on the I CARE Advisory Board. He has served as Louisiana State Medical Society Governor's appointee to the Addictive Disorders Resource Authority and to the Child Death Investigation Review Board.

Dr. Cataldie has served as Medical Director of the Louisiana State Board of Nursing and is currently an addictionologist for the Board's Recovery Nurse Program. He is the Medical Director of the Physician's Health Foundation of Louisiana.

His current addictionology practice also includes providing detoxification, evaluation, and treatment on both an inpatient and outpatient basis for people wishing to recovery from the brain disease of addiction.

Informal Biographical Sketch

Formal Biographical Sketches don't really tell you much about a person. For that reason, I've decided to insert an informal "sketch" here in case you want to know something about me and why I do what I do. On June 28, 1978, all of my attention was turned to the disease of addiction. And, over the past 35 years (Wow, that looks like a lot of years when I see it in print!), I have read whatever I could get my hands and eyes on about addictions. I am a voracious reader. It was somewhat of a challenge finding scientific information about this disease in the pre-internet days. Now there is almost too much data. Unfortunately, volume is not necessarily an indicator of value. I find lots of misinformation and even biased information "out there." (Be careful what you wish for, I guess.) Also, since late 1978, I have evaluated and/or treated over 10,000 people suffering from this brain disease. As an "emergency room physician" (there was no such thing as an Emergency Medical Specialty at the time), I am sure I treated many addicts before my "addiction awareness epiphany", I just did not know it. I had blinders on until that fateful day when my attorney guided me to the nurse's station in the Chemical Dependency Unit in the hospital where I worked and told me I needed to stay there. He was right. Great guy! Thank you for being there, Chip.

In 1978, everyone in the addiction field was still talking about the "disease concept." Addiction was sort of a nebulous entity. Now, with all the brain, genetic, epigenetic, and addiction research, we properly talk about "the brain disease of addiction." In '78, you were lucky if you could even get a physician to come see a patient in a treatment facility. Now, we have Addictionologists; however, there is still a shortage.

We have made great strides in identifying and treating this

deadly brain disease, but before we all start patting ourselves on the back, let us take note of the fact that only ten percent of the people with this illness ever get treatment. Treatment is a gift. You might not see it that way at first, but if you are an addict reading this, you are probably one of that fortunate ten percent.

I think it is appropriate to provide you with a little insight into how I developed my writing style, especially since I am asking you to subject yourself to it. Admittedly, it is a rather informal style. I was "raised up" in a family riddled by alcoholism. Thankfully, there were two very wonderful people in my life who gave me the tools that I would later need when my "house of cards" collapsed in '78. I had a very pragmatic Hard Shell Baptist grandmother who lived up in the piney woods at a place called "Breezy Hill." There was no TV there. Actually, there was no running water there either, and she cooked on a wood-burning stove. Yes, that is true. So, what does one do in the evening when there is no TV? One sits down with his grandmother, and they read the bible out loud to each other. That's what.

The other wonderful person was her counterpart, namely, my very Roman Catholic grandmother. When I stayed with her, she made sure I was perched in a pew on every possible occasion. I was not fond of being made to go to church, but I did not get to vote. Still, I always liked that part of the mass where the priest would read a parable. If I could visualize stuff, I could understand it better.

I share all this because I tend to write like I think and talk.

My sixth-grade grammar teacher, Ms. Normand, encouraged that style and it stuck. For the record, any "stories" or scenarios I use in this book are based on reality but not on any one person, unless I am sharing information about my own addiction. There is no violation of anyone's confidentiality. If you see yourself or someone else in a scenario, it is only because people with this disease exhibit similar signs and symptoms.

Additionally, I think it is germane to state what this publication is not. It is not a formal scientific medical research paper. You won't find footnotes and lists of references in the back of it. This is a compilation of knowledge I have gleaned from years of reading, research, and teaching. (I do love to teach.) More importantly, it is a compilation of my experiences in this field. It is about a chronic, progressive, and destructive (but treatable) brain disease. It's written because so many people in recovery or people just entering recovery or people treating addicts or people living with addicts ask me about this topic all the time. (Well, not all the time but frequently; sorry, Ms. Normand).

This disease is about people and that is why I present this information to you. It is my hope that this helps answer some of your questions about the people you are and the people you care about and the people who care about you. It is my hope that this journalistic effort may offer some guidance and solace to those of you who are on the bittersweet journey of getting sober.

TABLE OF CONTENTS

Science Meets Common Sense

"Enquiring minds want to know." That was or is the motto of the *National Enquirer*, a gossip tabloid that my mother was addicted to (among other things like alcohol and drugs). She hoarded back issues of that rag all her life. There are two things I remember from the *Enquirer*: "Bat Boy" and that motto which became my mantra of sorts.

My inquiring mind centers on addiction. There are a couple of reasons for this. I happen to have this brain disease which has been in remission for 36 years. That in and of itself is reason enough to learn everything I can about it. However, I also find this brain disease to be absolutely fascinating.

The field of addictionology is exploding with new information. Mountains of scientific information are being generated on addictions, and there are avalanches of data cascading down them every day. But what good is an avalanche of research information to you if it's tucked away in esoteric scientific journals?

I wrote this book because I want to sort out this information and present it to my patients and others who are interested in addictions. The more you know about your disease, the better you are prepared "to do what you need to do" to get well and stay that way. Knowledge is not power, but knowledge plus action is power. Accurate knowledge can empower you to take appropriate action. Of course, inaccurate "knowledge" can lead you to take inappropriate action and get worse.

My self-imposed task is to bring applicable scientific information into the real world so that you and I can use it to help ourselves and others. In short, if you are an alcoholic/addict, I want you to know about your disease, and I want you to recover. I learn more about this disease every day by reading about it, treating it, and having it. However, I must admit that I was not always a willing student when it came to addictions.

When I "bottomed out" and entered treatment at the behest of the judge, I was more than skeptical of the whole recovery process. I did not enter treatment to get into recovery. I entered treatment to get out of jail. I figured I could do "my time" in a nice treatment center which would get the heat off me, and then I could go about my business as usual.

Much to my dismay, I found myself trapped in the midst of what I discounted as a bunch of "Big Book thumping AA fanatics." But, hey, it beat two bologna sandwiches twice a day, if you know what I mean, so I settled in and started counting days.

Then one morning, the cult leader, who called himself my counselor, announced we were having a "Big Book" study. My first thought was "here comes more indoctrination." Per usual, I readied my rigid, addicted mind to resist whatever this "counselor" had to say. My only hope was that we would get through the obligatory programming in time for me to be first in the lunch line. The lesson of the day was called "the promises." That word "promises" made me flinch. My sarcastic thought was they would soon be offering a magical prayer cloth for us to purchase. I mumbled a litany of profanities under my breath as I acquiesced to reading the section de jour.

Then "lo and behold," as I read about those promises, I found hope. This recovery stuff was starting to make sense even to my foggy mind. It was then that I fearfully put aside my mantle of cynicism and decided to give it a try. It worked. Those promises that I secretly and desperately wanted gradually came true for me, and they still do today.

I need to insert a disclaimer here since I am making reference to information printed in the "Big Book" of Alcoholics Anonymous (AA). I do not represent or speak for AA in any way, shape, form, or manner. You can find the original promises in the book <u>Alcoholics Anonymous</u>.

I think AA is a good way to recover. It helped me. But, as you will see in the section under treatment options, I do not think AA is the only way to recover. One really good thing about AA is that you can take it or leave it. That alone kills the cult theory. There are no AA police persons, albeit there may be police persons in AA.

At the time of my first "Big Book" study, I scribbled a few cryptic words onto my book's margins. This was definitely a turning point for me. As part of my preparation for this book, I reviewed those notations that were written by a then shaky hand which I had attributed to a familial tremor. By the way, that "familial tremor" went away when I stopped using as did that familial high blood pressure. That aside, I want to share my reflections on those words that I jotted down so feverishly lest I would forget them at the time. I share them with all my patients and have done so for thirty-plus years. Here they are:

"Break free": If you are an addict, you are shackled to your compulsions and your pain. You might remember what happiness is, but you are insulated from feeling it now by your sick, addicted brain. You would like to feel some real happiness again, but you're trapped and your way is not working. I have great news. You can break free of the chains. You can reclaim your high jacked brain. You can experience real happiness. I've done it. I've seen others do it. It requires putting aside false pride and false humility. It requires learning to think from the top down like functional people

instead of from the bottom up like some mammal scurrying in a sewer. In short, it requires being human.

"Clean Slate": What I longed for the most was the proverbial "clean slate." Recovery is the chance to start over and leave the garbage behind. We addicts accumulate a lot of garbage. Many is the addict who would like to just forget it all. Well, news flash, you can't forget it so good luck on that. The only option available, if you want out of your addiction, is to deal with the past. If you don't deal with it, it will deal with you and control you. You can learn from the past or you can get stuck in it. With help, you can go through the shame and the guilt of your past and come out with a different view of life and different goals. You can get back in sync with your values, have self-worth, have real pride, and be an asset rather than a liability. You can get your healthy brain circuits working and override the pathological circuits of addiction. When you achieve this, you will have choices and empowerment to make your own decisions rather than being manipulated by a pathological addict brain that has only one concern: getting the next drink, pill, or powder. One of the most common fears I hear from addicts when we talk about this aspect of recovery is, "Yeah, but what if I screw it up again?" This self-defeating statement is "addict-brain thinking." If you develop your healthy brain circuits and exercise them, you don't have to screw up again. If you do screw up, you don't have to stay screwed up.

"Anxiety/Fear": Most of us addicts live in a state of anxiety and fear. We get anxiety from many sources. Some of us may have been born with anxiety, and we made it worse with alcohol and or other drugs, usually much worse. We also get anxiety from the brain damage we are perpetuating with each drug intake. Then there is the fear of getting caught doing any or all addict behavior. You know the behaviors: lying, cheating, stealing, hiding, committing crimes, violating personal and family values, etc., etc. Plus,

there is that internal conflict and worry. Living with "free floating" anxiety 24/7 is going to lead you into a relapse and subsequently into more anxiety.

Your anxiety isn't going to miraculously go away, but you can find peace in "doing the right thing," and you can learn techniques such as stress management to deal with it. If you need medications for anxiety, you can work with a professional to get the ones you need as opposed to the ones your addicted brain wants.

"Self-Pity": Addicts tend to "wallow in self-pity like hogs in slop." (You can blame that idiom on my grandfather who worked a 40-acre farm in North Louisiana.) We load ourselves up with negative self-thoughts and negative self-perceptions and even self-loathing, and then we actually use all that to dive back into the slop of addiction. That brings on more consequences and more guilt and more shame, so we push others farther away. Then we wallow in more self-pity like hogs in slop and then we get more consequences and the cycle goes on and on and the slop gets deeper and deeper. If you get tired of living in slop, there is a way out.

Addicts are self-centered and think the world revolves around their own infantile need to feel the continued effects of drugs on the damaged reward centers in their brains. Addicts build walls of self-serving attitudes and behaviors. Then they get angry when someone challenges these rigid drug-serving defenses. If you are an active addict, everything (and I mean "everything") is less important than putting that drug into your addict brain. You might not see it that way, but everyone else does. One of the main things wrong with that damaged brain of yours is that it does not know what is wrong with it. The natural progression of this self-centeredness is to ultimately drive away everyone who really cares for you or even has the capacity to really care for you. The end result is isolation and loneliness. We can change that. Addiction might not be a choice, but recovery is.

Donna

Donna is 21-years-old and mature well beyond her years if you can call what I am seeing maturity. She thinks it is. She is wrong. She has plenty of life experiences. Many of these experiences should be reserved for someone at least ten years older; however, many of them should not be experienced by anyone at all. She went from childhood into a brief adolescence that was cut short by her drug use and is now talking like she's a grown woman. I guess she is in some superficial aspects.

She's attractive, which is somewhat of a curse that I hope we can help her turn into a blessing. She obviously has some innate intelligence, but she has been busy underachieving lately. How do I know that? Well, for one thing she's sitting in my office in a residential treatment center for drug addiction. I don't think her initial goal in life was to become an addict.

As we pick our way along the road of her drug history, she relates an all-too-familiar story. She has little idea as to what she is really telling me or that her words are being filtered through eyes and ears that have been seeing and hearing versions of this same story for over a third of a century. It occurs to me that I have been treating addictions longer than she has been alive. Unfortunately, it may be longer than she lives to be if she keeps it up. I do have hope that she can "get into recovery" because other members of her family have done so. I treated Donna's mother when she was an adolescent. I hope no one will have to treat Donna's daughter.

> *"I started drinking at 13 years old. Yeah, that's also about the time I tried my first cigarette. It made me so dizzy at first, but I did it again and again. Now I smoke about a half pack to a pack a*

day. I smoke more when I use opiates, of course. It was the same thing with marijuana. I tried it at 13 or 14, and I didn't really like it that much at first. I guess I really started drinking and using at about 15 or 16. Then my boyfriend had some Roxies so I tried that. I liked it but I just used it to party, but it got to be a habit and I got in trouble, so here I am."

Donna's very first statement here is most profound, albeit she probably doesn't know it. *"I started drinking at 13 years old."* I'm no longer seeing an attractive young woman before me. My mind's eye has dissected its way into her brain, and I am assessing her neural pathways. I see those circuits that drive us to achieve. Hers are crippled. Drug use has distorted her basic ability to seek and repeat healthy behaviors. I see frontal lobes that have been under assault by drugs for eight critical years. These lobes sit right behind the front of her skull. These lobes are for making decisions, weighing options, delaying gratification, planning for the future, and projecting who we are onto the world. I'm listening to a 21-year-old woman whose decisions are powered by the frontal lobes of a twelve-year-old child. I see a mess - a hard-wired mess. One of the things wrong with this brain is that it really does not know what is wrong with it.

"My mom is overprotective and she over-reacts. She used to have a drug problem so anyone who drinks or takes anything is an addict in her eyes. I'm not my mom. At least my dad doesn't go around judging me. I mean, yeah, he was mad when I got arrested, but he didn't let me sit in jail like my mom wanted him to. I guess I have to move in with them when I get out of here. That should really suck, but don't tell them that!"

Donna thinks she has her mom and dad figured out and compartmentalized into their own little boxes. Mom doesn't understand her and dad rescues her. She discounts mom for having the very thing she desperately needs – recovery. When the proverbial fan gets saturated and is spraying the mess about, she does her rendition of "daddy's little helpless girl" and tries to play her dad like a fiddle. Evidently it worked this time, he bailed her out.

> "Why am I here? I'll be honest with you. I had to come here because my lawyer said it would help with my case. I think they are going to make some sort of deal. I'll probably end up in drug court or something. I mean big deal - all I had was a few Roxies and a syringe. That stuff wasn't even mine. I guess my boyfriend stuck it under the seat or something. I am not really worried about all that."

Apparently, Donna thinks she also has the legal system figured out. She thinks she will go through the motions here while her parents pay for a lawyer, and she will get a slap on the wrist for committing a felony. She thinks she is bulletproof.

> "I was waiting tables. Well, yes, there were lots of drugs there. There was lots of cash too. Anyway, I'm going to go back to school. I'm thinking about being a nurse. I went to college for a year, but I was partying too much and missing classes and my grades were bad, so I dropped out for a while. My mom was really pissed; sorry I mean angry, about that because I lost my financial aid - but she got over it. Anyway, I can go back to waiting tables and get the money for college."

She even has society figured out. I will not challenge all that addict-skewed thinking right now. Nursing Boards do background checks and demand disclosure of any addiction treatment. You don't just waltz in. I remind myself that this is a twelve-year-old brain I am talking to.

Her odds on getting sober the first time out are not good. That doesn't mean we are not going to try. It means the odds are against her. If we plant some seeds of hope, she may come around this time or the next or the next. One strong predictor of success is the level of motivation a person has to recover. Donna's only motivation right now is to "do her time" here in treatment and get "relief" of the latest consequence of her addiction. (I can relate.)

Maybe we can begin to correct the mis-wiring in her brain and help her become grounded in reality. Make no mistake; she is the most critical person on the team, but right now she is more interested in playing us than working with us.

It will take her brain at least two years of being drug free to reach a "normal" state. I assure you she is not ready to hear that right now let alone begin to internalize it. She couldn't process it even if she were willing because her brain is diseased and acutely toxic. She has sensitized her brain to chemicals. She has an allergy to them. If she uses, she reactivates the whole neurological chain of events immediately. There is no time off for good behavior. It is a disease! An addicted brain never forgets how to handle mood-altering chemicals. It does so badly. If she smokes cigarettes, she increases her odds for relapse. If she smokes, I question whether or not she is in recovery. Let me correct that: if she smokes, she is not in recovery. If she smokes, we are no longer talking recovery, we are talking degrees of consequences. Cigarette addiction results in long-term consequences. Opiate addiction has more immediate ones.

> *My drug of choice? I like opiates. I do three or five*
> *Roxies a day. I used to snort them. I never*

thought I would do IV. I'm afraid of needles. Yeah, I have shared but only with my boyfriend. He's clean. Cotton fever? Yeah, I had that a couple of times. It's a bitch. I don't think I really need treatment, I can stop on my own, but WTF, here I am. My last use? It was on the way here.

Heroin? Sure, I've tried it. We use that when we can't get Roxies. Lots of my friends are switching over to it.

Nope! No problem with anything else. We smoke weed every day but so what? It's only weed. I may do a bar (Xanax) now and then. Don't really drink. I have a prescription for Adderall, but I guess I can't take that here, huh? (She smiles.)

It would appear that Donna has it all figured out, including me. Donna is "in control." Well, as in control as Captain Edward John Smith, the captain of the Titanic, and it's full steam ahead or downward, as the case may be.

It doesn't take a psychic to predict her future: a life of manipulating and being manipulated, physical and emotional abuse, a series of failed relationships, a litany of failed expectations, various pregnancies with undetermined outcomes, physical illnesses, maybe some Hepatitis C, maybe some venereal disease, perhaps some chronic pain along the way, some legal issues related to criminal activity or civil matters such as divorce and child custody, depression, anxiety, and misery masked by drugs and the quest for self-worth through materialism and seeking the approval of various other people. All this tragic drama will continue until she is used up and has settled for a life that even reality TV will shy away from. She is sitting here before me with her diseased brain running the show, and she does not have any idea as to what she is really saying or where her life is headed.

Donna is clueless.

But, her makeup is perfect.

It's A Brain Disease

The brain disease of addiction is characterized by the compulsive and continued use of a mood-altering chemical or chemicals despite recurring adverse consequences.

If you are an alcoholic and/or addict or if you are married to one, engaged to one, in love with one, love one, or have one in your family or if you have kids, or responsible for kids or if you treat alcoholics and addicts, you need to know about the many risk factors involved in this brain disease. In fact, in our society where alcohol, cigarette tobacco, tobacco, and in some cases marijuana are legal, everyone needs to know about the risks.

These risk factors can be biological, psychological, and/or social. Some of the biological factors include genetics or even gender. Psychological risks include decision-making styles and how one views and interacts with the world. Prenatal experiences can impact the development of mood disorders and mental illness. Emotional and/or physical abuse can cause lasting physiological brain abnormalities and psychological consequences that predispose one to addiction. Social factors such as parenting and age at first use of a mood-altering substance definitely impact the risks of developing a substance-use disorder. To make things even more complicated, combinations of any of the above factors impact risk for addiction.

Most addicts start developing the brain disease of addiction before they are twenty-one years old. Why? Because most of them try mood-altering chemicals before the age of twenty-one and their brains are not fully developed and are therefore more vulnerable to the effects of such substances. A basic truism or axiom of addiction is: "the younger the user, the greater the damage." This is so blatantly obvious that it is common sense, right? Right! But common sense and addiction are like oil and water; they just don't seem to mix well.

Continued use of addictive drugs is accompanied by pathological brain changes that stick around even when the person is no longer using. In order for the addicted brain to recover, these pathological circuits must be overridden by healthy ones. Developing and maintaining healthy circuits is what recovery is all about.

To understand the pathologically addicted brain, or the "unwell" brain, one must first understand the functional or "well" brain. The developing brain has a normal route or "trajectory" that, if followed, results in the development of a functional, adaptive brain.

There are several stages to this normal developmental trajectory. Our brain grows from the bottom up. That means the basic survival parts grow first and promote functions like eating, drinking, seeking shelter, having sex, and other survival behaviors to assure success for the individual and the species. Some people call this lower-developed survival brain the "reptile brain." After that, we develop the higher functions like thinking capabilities. The last areas to develop are the frontal lobes. These lobes are responsible for "executive functions" such as decision making, reasoning, and social appropriateness. This higher functioning, or upper brain, is what makes us human.

During the development process, there is a time when we have an overabundance of nerve connections or synapses. Yep. We actually have too much brain tissue. You can envision the excess connections as being duplicate or redundant connections. You can also envision some as simply not being used. Plus, some of them are unhealthy. This surplus of connections triggers the brain to "select out" and keep the ones that are needed and get rid of the ones that are not needed. This selection process is critical, and which connections will stay and which will go away are determined primarily by what the brain experiences. The brain gets rid of the unneeded circuits and connections by a process called auto-pruning. The brain will selectively keep the connections and circuits that it has learned will lead to a "reward." The brain becomes wired to match rewarding experiences encountered during development. To get at the basic idea of how this works, we can take a look at my brain development as I approached the age of two years old.

> If we get hungry, we try to eat something. Toddlers taste all sorts of things. That first taste of something new is a trial run. If I eat ice cream, I get a reward. Mmm, ice cream good! My brain will want me to do that behavior again, so it wires me to eat ice cream. It may even develop different connections and circuits to furnish me with different ways to get my ice cream. The more I use those circuits to get ice cream, the stronger those circuits become.

> But, if I'm hungry and I bite the tail of the family cat, I get an adverse consequence that I would rather not repeat. Ugh, biting cat's tail not good! Cat tail biting did not activate my reward circuits. In fact it did just the opposite. Therefore, my brain is not going to develop or reinforce a circuit that promotes cat tail-biting. As such, the brain circuits that prompted that behavior will be pruned away, and I will not be motivated to bite the cat's tail again.

This amusing little one dimensional example of how I discovered ice cream illustrates how the "selective pruning process" will attempt to preserve and strengthen reward circuits. I still like ice cream to this day.

The selective pruning process will also attempt to eliminate unrewarding behaviors by eliminating unhealthy circuits. I have not bitten my cat's tail since I was two years old.

It also demonstrates that this learning and pruning process is based upon experience. Eating tasty food is a rewarding experience. Neurological pruning is aimed at molding goal-directed behaviors that will prompt me to re-experience that feeling. However, as we noted, this is a one dimensional example. Other circuits will develop to influence my ice cream eating behaviors so that I don't eat four gallons of the stuff a day.

The developmental processes and the learning curves associated with experience go far beyond the quest to get more ice cream. These processes are happening at all levels – biological, psychological, social, and spiritual – and are uniquely interwoven with extreme complexity into the inner being of the individual person.

This ultra-critical developmental process relies heavily, but not totally, upon parental guidance. I am not just learning about ice cream and cat tails here. I am molding a foundation for survival based largely upon what family values I experience and the associated good feelings I get from being in sync with those values.

If achievement is rewarded, I want to find a way to achieve, such as making good grades. In order to experience the reward associated with reaching that family value, I need brain circuits that will allow me to achieve good grades. This takes effort on my part.

If manners are important, I want to develop them.

If stealing is rewarded, I want to be a good thief, and I will develop those circuits.

If drug use is acceptable, I will develop circuits to become an addict.

If I live in a chaotic family, I may end up with chaotic circuits.

If I am exposed to stimuli that result in development of pathological circuits, this does not excuse my behavior. I am ultimately responsible for my own behavior. An explanation does not equate to an excuse. We will have more on this later.

After the pruning process, the remaining nerve transmission circuits become insulated or myelinated to enhance the efficiency of transmitting signals. In essence, the brain has "hard wired" itself.

Much of our brain developmental trajectory is guided by a host of chemicals within the brain as well as from the rest of the body. These include dopamine, serotonin, natural cannabinoids, GABA, glutamate, hormones, and too many more to mention. In addition to this, there are undoubtedly some brain molding or modeling chemicals that we do not even know about yet.

These internal chemicals respond to the environment and thereby guide development tailored to that environment. If drugs that act on the nervous system are taken into the body from the outside, these drugs can alter the normal balance of the critical internal chemicals. This can alter perception of the environment and thereby alter brain trajectory. Your brain can be mis-wired if you use alcohol and/or other drugs during this developmental process. Mis-wiring equals mental illness.

Developmental trajectory starts on <u>day one</u> of our existence and continues at some level throughout our entire lives. We all know that we started out as one cell, but you may not know that we stayed that way for only about a day. Then we started to sprout other cells, and you and I became a little ball of cells for a short while. We continued to make more and more of ourselves, and after about two weeks we had set down the foundation for the development of a brain and spinal cord. That foundation is called a neural plate. When all this was going on, we definitely did not need any outside chemicals coming in to interfere with and/or alter our development.

Unfortunately, that interference can start prior to anyone knowing we are around yet. Let us take a moment to consider the following scenario.

> *Mary got out of treatment three months ago. She met this "cool guy" at a twelve-step meeting, and they fell in lust. Both relapsed shortly thereafter. Today, she decided to get back into treatment. She missed her menstrual period, but that is not unusual given the fact that she started shooting heroin again about three weeks ago. "I got right back up to a half gram or more of heroin a day." Historically when she does heroin her periods are irregular. Her pregnancy test is positive.*
>
> *"Are you sure?" she says with a worried brow.*
>
> *"I'm sure. We ran it three times."*
>
> *"Have I harmed my baby?"*
>
> *The answer is: "I don't know. But I must inform you that you now have what doctors call a 'high*

risk pregnancy'. "

If Mary happens to be your mother, here is what you have been experiencing for the past twenty-one days. Not only have you have been floating in an opiate bath, you have also been getting a toxic load from your mother's cigarette smoking. Many women do not know they are pregnant in the early weeks of pregnancy, even when they are trying to get pregnant. By definition, not knowing is always the case if the pregnancy is unplanned. This was unplanned.

So what is the result of this toxic exposure? That's another unknown. What we do know is that at the fourth week of development, you are making brain cells (neurons) at the rate of 250,000 cells every minute. We also know that continued drug use on the part of your mother equals continued damage. Stopping as soon as possible will minimize any outside chemical interference in the developmental process.

Actually, the latest research verifies what anyone with a modicum of common sense already knows. The baby is better off if both mom and dad stop using for months before conceiving a child.

Some substances are more poisonous or neurotoxic to the brain than others. The use of "synthetic marijuana" may have detrimental effects on brain development as early as two weeks into the pregnancy. The operative phase is "may have detrimental effects." Animal studies indicate "synthetic weed" poses a significant danger of damage to the developing brain. We will talk about other drugs and specific maldevelopments, such as fetal alcohol syndrome, in a later section.

Fortunately, many female addicts stop using everything during pregnancy. When I ask them about why they stopped, the answer put forth is very simple: "It was not fair of me to harm my baby." Unfortunately, many start up again shortly after birth. While I commend mom for not using during pregnancy, I am very concerned that resuming an active addiction once the baby is born is going to harm the child in other ways. Children, especially newborns, need sober moms. Sadly, I have witnessed this relapse phenomenon many times also.

There is another sad truth. About 15% of pregnant addicts do not stop using. Most are ambivalent about using during pregnancy, and many tell me they tried to stop. Some just have personality disorders or are so steeped in their addiction that they cannot or will not stop using. Some who continue to use tell me they used during previous pregnancies and the baby came out okay. By okay, that means the child looked okay. The ravages of impaired brain development due to mom's drug use during pregnancy may not be apparent for years to come.

Once a pregnant addict decides to stop using, she would be ill-advised to stop abruptly or go "cold turkey." Detox during pregnancy can be complex and complicated, and mom and fetus need a controlled medical detoxification for lots of reasons that affect them both mutually and independently.

There is another point that is very relevant to our current scenario. If Mary was your mom, you may have been programmed to be an addict while you were the size of a watermelon seed. However, just because you may have been programmed for a high risk of addiction, does not mean you are going to be an addict and is not an excuse to become an addict, and it is definitely not an excuse to stay an addict. Addictive brain disease is like any other disease with a genetic risk. There are many variables. These variables are often grouped under two broad headings called nature which refers to genetics and nurture which refers to the environment you are raised in.

Let's say you have a family history of heart disease. Specifically, let's say your uncle and your father both ended up with heart attacks due to clogged heart arteries or coronary artery disease at about age thirty five years old. Both required coronary artery bypass surgery. Does that mean you are going to have a heart attack at that age? Maybe or maybe not! A lot depends on you. If you are eighty pounds overweight, lie on the couch eight hours a day, eat hog cracklings all day long, never exercise except to waddle back and forth to the fridge for a half gallon of Blue Bell at a time, then you are high risk for getting a surgical scar on your chest. If you eat and exercise properly, do not smoke, and take medication that keeps your cholesterol down, you decrease your risk.

For example, let us say you have a family history of addictive brain disease. Let's get even more specific and say you have a family history of alcoholism. Your uncle and your father both ended up in jail due to multiple DUIs at around age thirty-five years old. Does that mean you are going to have a steady diet of green bologna sandwiches and wear an orange jumpsuit while picking up garbage on the side of the highway? Maybe it does or maybe it does not! A lot depends on you and your behaviors. If you are glugging down a 6 pack of beer on the way home from work because that's what Uncle Joe taught you to do, you are at high risk for alcohol dependency. Moreover, if you are in a bar with your drinking buddies wondering if your wife has taken the kids and left because she says you drink too much, you've already joined the team. Even at that stage of your alcoholism, you may not really think you are an alcoholic. Sounds crazy? That's because it is crazy. It is the insanity of the addicted brain.

An addiction is not activated until you put the mood-altering chemicals into your brain. If you never drink, you can never become an alcoholic. Also, if you wait until you have a fully developed brain and you drink, your risk of becoming dependent is greatly reduced. If you have a family history of addictive brain diseases, you should give strong consideration to avoiding addictive substances altogether.

Having said all that, let us get back on track as to how this brain disease develops. We have already noted that your mother's experiences with alcohol and or other drugs during pregnancy can impact your brain development. Actually, any major stressors that mom experiences can impact your brain adversely as can her nutritional intake. Prescribed drugs such as mood stabilizers and antidepressants can also have adverse effects on you.

As an aside, it is amazing to me how little some people know about their own prenatal histories. I often get a blank stare when I ask a patient about this – especially some of the guys. If you do not know about your prenatal history, I encourage you to ask.

Once you are born into the world and start growing up, there are events beyond your control that can promote the development of an addictive brain. These events include stressors such as child abuse, family discord, social issues, co-existing brain issues such as ADHD, anxiety, depression, and a host of other things.

The greatest predictor of developing an addictive brain disease is the age at which the person first used a mood-altering substance. The most vulnerable time to start becoming an addict is in adolescence.

A developing adolescent brain is still relying heavily on its reward systems to let it know if it is doing the right things. If you do the right thing, you get a boost to the reward center and you feel good. To succeed in life, we need that reward center to activate when we do positive things, such as making an "A" on a test, getting that coveted part in the school play, or hitting a home run. In short, that boost lets us know we are achieving worthy accomplishments. It is also necessary for survival of self and species. That same reward center goes off when we eat tasty food. Can you imagine what would happen if eating did not feel good? You could conceivably starve to death. It is rewarding to fall in love and to have children, and it is rewarding to reach a spiritual awareness.

Our brain reward systems serve to guide us toward healthy goal-directed behaviors – like choosing a career path or even a mate. All sorts of complex brain functions are tied to these decisions. For instance, in order to make appropriate decisions, you must have good frontal lobe function. You must be able to socialize appropriately. You must have an intact memory system. And you must be able to learn from successes as well as mistakes. In the adolescent brain, the reward system is wide open and wanting to try new things, but the frontal lobes are not fully developed. In other words, the throttle is wide open, but the brakes are not working well. This creates a time frame that is both opportune and dangerous.

The danger is that the reward circuits that exist to guide you to achieve your potential can be hijacked by the use of mood-altering drugs. After all, if you can take a drug and have your reward systems light up right away, why should you bother to do all that other stuff that requires so much effort to achieve? This is the addiction trap. With time, the use of substances overrides all sources of natural rewards, and then the drug owns you.

This can happen to adults as well as to adolescents. I have

treated several adults who did not get addicted until exposed to prescription medications that were prescribed for legitimate reasons.

"I don't consider myself an addict like these other people. I have never even seen a marijuana cigarette or heroin, and I would not even know how to use it. It would scare me to death to be around it. It's illegal and I've seen what it can do. My brother is a drug addict and an alcoholic. He is in a jail right now. My husband and I do not smoke or drink. We are both active in our church. This all started when I got in this wreck about four years ago, and I got rear-ended and got ruptured discs in my back. I went to my doctor for a while; then she sent me to a pain clinic, but they kicked me out last week because I was using too much medicine and getting some pain pills from other places. They make you sign a contract, you know. I admit that at first the pills made me feel good. The medicine stopped my pain, but it also stopped my depression, and it gave me energy to do my housework and my chores. We own and work a farm. It's a hard life, but we would not have it any other way. I have been taking more and more to get me going. I can't even get out of bed without taking a couple of pills. I put them on the night stand every night. It is the first thing I do in the morning. I have been getting real sick since they stopped my medicine. I got some of my daddy's pills from my momma and bought some more from a friend. My husband actually paid for them. He's very worried about all this and is very angry at the doctors, but it is my fault. I have been getting them from other places, too. The pills just took over and I let it happen. I can take up to ten or fifteen Lortabs a day. My regular doctor sent me here. This is the only place we have to turn to. I am really scared and ashamed and

nervous." Carol, onset of addiction, age forty-one years old.

Carol is an adult onset addict. She had a genetic predisposition to become addicted. This is one of the reasons it is so important for a doctor to know what diseases run in your family. If several people in your family are allergic to penicillin, I need you to tell me that. I would be concerned that you might also be prone to that allergy, and I would think about prescribing a different antibiotic or at least monitoring you really closely if I prescribed it to you. If the disease of brain addiction runs in your family, I would be very cautious about prescribing an addictive drug like Lortab. If you needed it, I would caution you about the added genetic risk of taking it and would monitor your use. Addiction can be an insidious process. It sneaks up on you.

In Carol's case, I would argue that this is, in part, an iatrogenic addiction. Iatrogenic means the problem is caused by the physician (or other prescriber) and is due to the treatment he or she rendered to the patient. Iatrogenic addiction is nothing new. As a matter of historical reference, over 2300 years ago, a royal physician by the name of Erasistratus warned against this very thing when he declared that "opium should be completely avoided" ostensibly due to the risk of dependency.

There was also a Greek philosopher by the name of Diagoras who stated over 1700 years ago that it was better to suffer pain rather than take opium and become dependent upon it.

Opiate addiction and related problems including iatrogenic dependency have been with us a long time.

For clarity, I am not saying Carol does not have a degree of responsibility in the process. I am saying she has a physiological brain disease and needs an evaluation and detoxification to see where we go from here.

Prognosis: The pathology of brain addiction is progressive but not necessarily in a linear manner. Some times are better than others. For instance, there may be moments of clarity and periods of abstinence. If left unabated, this brain disease will progress. It tends to progress at different rates in different people depending upon the individual, the situation, and even the addictive substance; however, the brain disease of addiction definitely gets worse with ongoing drug use.

The progression can be halted, and new healthy circuits can be developed. Unfortunately, some addicts do not get help until after they end up with lasting brain damage that does not correct fully. They must learn ways to compensate for such deficits. Healthy circuits must be exercised and maintained to avoid slipping back into pathological thinking. Recovery is an ongoing process but then again, so is life.

An Introduction to Treatment and Recovery

My father used to tell me a story and would laugh every time he told it, to, which seemingly was often and replete with more and more embellishments. Then again, he was a fifth-a-day man when he was "in his cups," and he may have been in a blackout on some of those occasions and subsequently may not have remembered telling it. At any rate, I remember it, and I'll share the short, unembellished version with you.

> *There is this guy who tries to take a shortcut from Shreveport to Alexandria, and he ends up lost and driving around the back roads of North Louisiana. He sees a local farmer and stops for directions on how to get to Alexandria. The farmer rubs his head and commences to give the city slicker directions. "Well you can go down Brown Road and hit the Kisatche Forest Fire Break road; nope you could never find it. Okay, you could go over to Butterman's Branch Road and turn north at the Kramer farm; nope, he might shoot you...This goes on for a while, and the farmer, somewhat exasperated turns to the city slicker and says, "**YOU** can't get there from here!" [Ha ha ha ha ha...]*

Not unlike our unfortunate driver, an addict cannot get to safety and escape from a catastrophic fate until he or she is grounded in reality and has the maps and tools to recover. For many addicts, those tools are found in "treatment."

So, what is treatment?

The answer may come as a surprise to you because 'treatment" is not adequately defined. Indeed, "treatment" is a very broad "catch-all term." Subsequently, there is really no agreed-upon standard of care for "treatment." There is also a general lack of requirements for those who offer treatment-including addiction counselors. I strongly encourage you to ask about credentials. Another problem we have with treatment is that outcome studies are sorely lacking.

When I hear the term treatment, I always ask, "What type?"

Likewise, when I hear the term therapist, I also inquire as to the type of therapist. There are state credentialing bodies that assure an appropriate level of skill and education, and there are national organizations that promote quality therapists. However, unless you are in the field, you probably would not know about all that. An addictionologist will know and would be a good place to start if you are looking for addiction treatment.

While this may sound pretty confusing at first glance, be assured that there is hope, and people do recover.

Although we don't have an official standard of care for treatment, we do have an official definition for "recovery." According to the Substance Abuse and Mental Health Services Administration (SAMHSA), **RECOVERY** is a process of change through which individuals improve their health and wellness, live a self-directed life, and strive to reach their full potential. Sounds simple enough, doesn't it? There's more to it, of course. There are four generalized areas of living that gauge recovery:

- **Health**: Taking responsibility for managing one's disease, and living a healthy life both emotionally, physically, and financially
- **Home**: Creating a safe and secure place to live
- **Purpose**: Participating in daily activities that provide a sense of purpose: volunteer work, school, job, family care-taking, art, or whatever gives you a sense

of fulfillment and accomplishment
- **Community**: Renewing or developing healthy relationships and social networking that give support, love, friendship, and hope

The "Ten Guiding Principles of Recovery" put forth by SAMHSA are worth reviewing and elaborating upon.

Hope – Hope is fostered by associating with peers in the recovery process. It is the feeling of knowing people can and do recover and so can you.

> *"When I walked into my first meeting, I was greeted by room full of people in recovery. People who wanted to help me into recovery also. It was a very powerful experience and made me realized that I was not alone in my struggle."* Tommy, 23-year-old heroin addict.

Person Driven – Ultimately treatment is self-determined and self-directed. Treatment provides a framework, but the individual must do the actual work, define individual recovery goals, and make informed decisions.

> *"The program is pretty simple, but the work is definitely not simple. Recovery is not a spectator event. Just sitting in a meeting is not going to get you well any more than just looking at a tool set is going to fix your car. You get out of it what you put into it."* As told to a newcomer by his sponsor who is 13 years sober.

Holistic – Recovery is a biological, psychological, social, and spiritual process. Subsequently, recovery requires an array of resources. Most addicts need help finding and using those resources. Hence, there is need for recovering peers, sponsors, therapists, family members, and others.

"I was in detox for five times over a two-year period. I kept going to detox and thinking that I would never drink again and that I had learned my lesson. I even detoxed in jail once. That was rough. I really figured I had learned my lesson after that. But, I went back and did the same thing over and over. I reached a new bottom when I picked up my third DWI. I finally surrendered to the fact that detox is not enough. I need the whole program." Kenny, alcoholic, 32 years old.

Peer and Allies – Mutual support is required. Loyalty and respect of the group members, social learning, and a feeling of belonging are all essential elements needed to free one's self of this addictive brain disease.

"It's great to be able to come here and talk to people who really understand. I mean, my family loves me, and all and they support me but they have no idea how powerful this compulsion can be and how my crazy mind tells me I might be able to use heroin again. But I know everybody in this room understands it and can help me get through my insanity." Carol, 23-year-old heroin addict, 3 months out of residential treatment.

Relationships and Social Networks – In order to engage in a life without drugs, the recovering addict needs family, friends, and healthy networks. Living a life of recovery is fulfilling and even fun, but isolation is a road to relapse.

"I knew she was going to relapse. All she did was feel sorry for herself because she couldn't use heroin anymore. She wouldn't go to family functions or engage in family activities. Her sponsor said she was "dry drunking," whatever that means. All I know is that she was miserable and seemed to want everyone

else to be miserable. She stopped going to NA and starting using even worse than before. We had to kick her out of the house again." Shelly's mom at an Al-Anon meeting.

Individual, Family, and Community Strengths – The individual has the personal responsibility to recover. No one else can do it for him or her. Families have responsibilities to help but there is a boundary between supporting an addict into recovery and enabling an addict to stay sick. The community shares the same burden. While drug diversion programs and drug court are most helpful, if the individual violates the recovery contract, legal consequences should follow.

"I know they do not play games in drug court. I relapsed over the weekend and I knew I was going test "hot" on the drug screen and then I was going to jail. I came here to treatment to stop using and get back into my program. I need to call and let them know where I am at. Maybe I can go to sober living instead of jail." James 20-year-old addict in drug court due to possession of schedule II drugs.

Culture and Influence – Culture and cultural background in all of its diverse representations including values, traditions, and beliefs—are keys in determining a person's journey and unique pathway to recovery.

"I wasn't sure I would fit in here, but I'm finding out this disease is an equalizer and we are all in the same boat. I feel accepted and I don't see anybody picking up the 'first stone.'" Cedric, 24-year-old synthetic marijuana addict.

Trauma – Trauma issues such as Post Traumatic Stress Disorder or PTSD must be addressed professionally and therapeutically as should any other co-existing disorder(s).

Recovery must offer a "safe place" to deal with such issues.

> *"I thought it was somehow wrong to talk about being raped by my uncle. I thought somehow it was my fault anyway, so I kept it a 'family' secret during my other treatments. I used Xanax to escape and numb me out. We all see how well that worked out. I am not going to be a victim anymore! I know this is a safe place, and I am talking about it this time and getting some relief."* Cheryl, Klonopin and Ambien addict, 26-years-old and in treatment for the third time.

Respect – This is another two-way street. I respect anyone trying sincerely to recover from this brain disease. It takes courage to "face those demons." I also expect that person to respect others. As a matter of fact, I believe this so much that if you are repeatedly disrespectful to others in the treatment program's community, I will invite you to leave.

Many Pathways – Recovery is not linear which means it does not follow a straight line of constant improvement. The journey of recovery is progressive, but it is often accompanied by "ups and downs." Treatment setbacks are a natural, but not inevitable, part of the process. You will hear the phrase "Progress not Perfection." It's a good one to embrace.

The right pathway to recovery is the one that works for you. There are many different approaches and modalities to addiction treatment that may prove to be a good fit. However, since there are many different treatment approaches available, it is important to know the common characteristics and components shared by the ones that actually work.

Components of Effective Treatment Programs – If you are in the market for an addictions' treatment provider, there are several things to look for. The first thing to do is find out what the treatment philosophy is for the facility. I believe addiction is a biological, psychological, social, and spiritual disease, and all of these essential life elements must be addressed to achieve a maximal level of recovery. As stated earlier, there is no agreed-upon standard for treatment. Therefore, not everyone agrees with this concept and not everyone deals with the components in the same manner, if at all.

> For instance, if I believe alcoholism is just a bad habit or a "learned behavior," I could devise a "treatment" (there's that word again) that would cure you. My treatment could make drinking alcohol such a horrible experience that you would never drink again. I could have a nice bar in my treatment facility and I could stock it with all sorts of "top shelf" booze. Then I could give you a drug that would make you sick as hell if you drink alcohol on top of it. Then I would make you drink at the bar. You would get sick every time I did this to you, and after a while the mere thought of an alcoholic drink or a bar would make you queasy so you would avoid drinking. This type of treatment really does exist, and it is called emetic (vomiting) aversion therapy. I don't recommend it as a course of therapy for lots of reasons not the least of which is that it addresses only one addictive drug, alcohol, and no other substances. I won't belabor the point, but I have not seen good outcome studies as to if it works. I know people who go through it may stay away from alcohol for a period of time, but is emetic therapy considered a success if you don't drink alcohol but you now take Valium on a regular basis? I think not. Let's not

throw the baby out with the bathwater. The medication (not the aversion process) does have a place in addiction treatment (more about that later).

I want to emphasize that although I believe certain components and principles are necessary for effective treatment, I do not believe a single type of treatment is right for everyone. I do not believe in "cookie cutter" therapy. Cookie cutter therapy is the process of trying to make one size fits all, and it can actually be harmful. I do not believe I can cram you into a mold and expect you to recover, or that one size fits all.

Here are some things to look for in a treatment program: (I put this in a quasi-checklist format so you can use it as a reference guide if you are talking to a prospective treatment center/program.)

- **Professional Staff:** This needs to include an addictionologist, psychologist, licensed addiction counselors, and knowledgeable, experienced nurses.
- **Outcome Studies:** You want to inquire as to how many people who get treatment there stay sober and for how long. You also want to know their definition of sobriety.
- **Comprehensive Assessment**: An individualized assessment and individualized treatment plan should be on the "front end" of treatment. Not all patients require the same approach.
- **Case Management:** A specific contact person, usually the patient's primary counselor, is needed as the main point of contact between the patient and any sources outside the program such as family members, employers, attorneys, and the like. This counselor must also encourage and monitor compliance in the treatment process. This therapist will also make sure

appropriate community assets are tapped into as part of the discharge plan.

- **Types of Therapy**: Group therapy, individual therapy, and family therapy are necessary and generally standard in any treatment setting. However, not all therapy is created equally. I encourage you to ask about how much of each will be forthcoming during treatment.

- **Social Skills Training:** Social interaction tends to suffer with addiction. Social skills training or re-training is best approached through cognitive behavioral therapy. CBT will address issues such as social anxiety, dealing with high relapse risk situations, interpersonal interactions, workplace issues, and the like.

- **Relapse Prevention Planning:** This is a must and should be a formalized process that equips the patients with an individualized, written plan to keep handy and refer to. Part of this plan can include "contingency contracting" which sets down what will happen should the person relapse.

- **Medications:** There are specific medications that are appropriate for some people with the brain disease of addiction. These medications cannot cure addictions but when clinically indicated, they can increase the effectiveness of other treatment interventions.

- **Specialized Services:** Treatment programs must be capable of assessing and addressing co-existing mental and/or medical diagnoses. Specialized services include gender specific groups, sexual trauma groups, healthcare professional groups, and other specialty groups for issues such as PTSD.

- **Duration of Treatment:** Primary treatment should last at least ninety days. The ninety days can be a combination of inpatient and outpatient, but the time from the day of admission until discharge into aftercare should be at least ninety days. Of course, when the potential patient hears this, it seems like an eternity. "OMG, I cannot do ninety days." Then again, most of my patients are coming into detox, and they cannot envision going two days without drugs let alone ninety days. For them, that is an eternity. This is one reason we do not force a commitment on them. We encourage them to forget about any time line right now, get safely detoxed, and then make an informed decision.

- **Continued Care**: This is also called "aftercare." Recovery is a process not an event. Recovery starts in treatment, but continued care is critical for ongoing freedom from active addiction. The longer one stays in a structured treatment setting, the greater the chances for a positive outcome. The addict needs to commit to at least a year of formal aftercare. Be sure and ask exactly what type of aftercare a facility provides. My bias is to have a therapist-run support group of twelve or so patients. Individual therapy and family therapy can be offered as needed.

- **Self-Help Groups:** Participation in support groups, such as Alcoholic Anonymous, is associated with better outcomes. That happens to be a fact. The question I frequently get is, "Why?" There is debate over why AA seems to work for some people and not others. Maybe the people who go to AA and benefit are just more motivated to change. Maybe this is a preselect group who can embrace the concept of a Higher Power. Maybe. I really do not have the answer. What I do have is advice to give it a try, and if it works for you, that is great news. If it works, "keep on keeping on." There are other mutual support groups, or self-help groups, that may also prove to be beneficial. I also know several people who got sober by going back or into church.

- **Motivational Therapy:** The stage of "motivation to change" is one of the strongest predictors of ongoing success in recovery. Motivational enhancement is part of any solid treatment program. (More on this later)

Barriers to Treatment – Unfortunately, just because there is good treatment, does not mean there is easy access to treatment. There are plenty of barriers – both external and internal.

The **stigma** of being an alcoholic or addict still exists. It is not as bad as it used to be but it is still there. However, the addict seems more attuned to "the stigma" than most of the general population. Most people really don't care that much and most realize recovery works. Addicts tend to focus on negatives, and they tend to do a lot of negative self-talk. Negative self-talk can lead to negative self-worth which in turn leads to negative self-fulfilling prophecies such as relapse.

> *"I worried for weeks about how people were going to treat me when I went back to work. I mean, I feel like I left there in disgrace. I have worked there as a nurse for seven years. Plus, the unit I work on is like an extended family, and I feel like I let them all down. I even thought about getting a job somewhere else rather than face them. But I managed to go back there, and I talked to my supervisor and a few of the other nurses, and they were just glad to have me back as my old self again. One of them even asked me how she could get her sister into recovery. I would have been a mistake for me to run from them. I would have kept running, from me."* Tammy, Registered Nurse in a Recovery Nurse Program, six months into sobriety.

Denial is the refusal or inability to see or accept the truth. Addicts tend to exhibit denial about their addictions.

Denial is rarely absolute; there are degrees of denial. For instance, I may think I have a problem but "it's under control" (minimizing). Addicts in denial deflect the reality of the seriousness of their brain dysfunction. As you recall, that is one of the things wrong with them. Their "haywire" brain circuits cause them to live in their own world of distorted reality. There are ways to "break through" that denial and give the addict a glimpse of reality which may prompt them to change. As a rule, direct confrontation of this denial does little good. There are "motivational counseling techniques" that are much more effective.

The **family** may also be in **denial.** Oftentimes the family adjusts itself to accommodate the addict. No parent wants to believe their child is an addict. The family has a wall of denial and defenses that unfortunately protect the addiction and enable the brain disease and its consequences to progress. Family members may "do the wrong things for the right reasons." Having to adjust the entire family system to accommodate an active addict requires a lot of time and energy on the part of other family members. It is very stressful living with an active addict, and that stress may impact the physical and mental health of other members, so much so, that another member may become the "identified patient" of a sick family system. Everybody loses. I have seen situations in which mom is hospitalized with a Major Depressive Disorder because she is at her "wit's end" and feels powerless over her twenty-three-year old addicted daughter who uses the grandbaby as a pawn to manipulate her mother and the entire family.

Some **employers** do **discriminate.** You won't find a sign out front saying "Addicts Need Not Apply." However, there are subtle ways to discriminate, and some employers do. The majority of employers do not discriminate; hence, the existence of Employee Assistance Programs and Professional Health Programs for doctors, dentists, nurses, pharmacists, psychologists, physician assistants, and other health care professionals. Obviously, it is best for the employee to come forward and use those services rather than be caught due to impairment on the job. When the latter happens, the situation goes from proactive to reactive. Then it is often a whole different game and generally not a good one.

Treatment can be very **expensive**. This is especially true if the addiction has caused a significant negative financial impact to the addict and his or her family. Addicts funnel money into their addictions to pay for drugs, legal fees, lawyers, doctors, and, in some cases, even gambling debts. That money may have been be meant for essential purposes, such as child support, rent, food, school supplies, etc. Most insurance companies cover addiction treatment to some degree; however, some do not. There is also the unfortunate occurrence that addicts have a tendency to get fired and lose insurance benefits.

Many **health care providers** are **not knowledgeable** about addictions and may miss the diagnosis and therefore delay getting the patient help.

The addict may **lack social support** because addictive behaviors drive others away. Addicts then gravitate towards dysfunctional social groups that revolve around alcohol and other drugs. When they do "bottom out," that dysfunctional group is a detriment, and at that point, the people who really care or cared about the addict may be totally alienated from him or her.

There may be **child custody issues,** and the addict fears going into treatment as this confirms he or she has a problem and is not a fit parent. This is truly impaired reasoning. It is usually not a secret that the person has a problem. If there is a custody battle going on, the issue is going to come to the surface. Seeking treatment shows motivation for positive change.

Child care may be an issue. Some programs assist with this factor.

The addict may not be able to comply with the **time commitment** needed for treatment. There are different levels of treatment. There is outpatient, intensive outpatient or partial hospitalization, in-patient, sober living houses, and a combination of all the above. Matching the person to treatment is important. I recommend the least restrictive level that circumstances permit.

Adverse legal issues (criminal and/or civil) may impede entering treatment. The person may have to do time in jail prior to entering a treatment program. Diversion programs, when appropriate are a good alternative to long-term incarceration, albeit there are times when a few days in jail can be a good motivator.

There may be legitimate **privacy concerns,** and there are circumstances in which it is best to "go away" for treatment. Upon return, the recovering addict needs to plug into an ongoing support system. Otherwise, he or she may be going away again and again.

<u>Formal Interventions</u> – An intervention is a very powerful process, the goal of which is to break through an addict's defenses and resistance to getting treatment for an addiction. It is a process that requires expertise, training, rehearsal, timing, and preparation. As with any powerful therapeutic tool, an intervention can also be a dangerous one. Choose your interventionist carefully!

In the early years of my recovery, I participated in several interventions based upon the Johnson Institute Model. The actual process consists of educating the family and/or concerned others about addiction and the associated pathological defenses the addict employs to protect his or her right to use addictive substances. The participants subsequently prepare a list of their concerns for the addict. They also list how the addict's behaviors impact them individually. Once this is accomplished, the trained interventionist reviews the information and a rehearsal is held. All possible reasons that the addict will give for not going to treatment or delaying treatment are anticipated. A treatment center is agreed upon and arrangements for admission are made prior to the intervention. This may even include having a court order ready for involuntary admission if the person refuses to comply. From there, a time and location is set for the intervention. The process is led by the interventionist, who lays down the ground rules to the addict and the process proceeds. The addict is counseled to listen to what these people who care have to say, and he or she will get an opportunity to respond once they have expressed their concerns and feelings. Each family member or concerned person then reads from his or her list. In essence, a mirror of the addictive behaviors and interpersonal consequences of addiction is being held up to the addict to reflect the severity of his or her brain disease. The goal is to get the addict some help. It usually works.

There are professional therapists who offer intervention services. As in choosing any health care professional, do your due diligence prior to signing on. Ask your physician about a referral, contact an addictionologist, and/or call a reputable treatment center. An intervention is powerful and dangerous. It creates a crisis for the addict even though it does so within a supportive environment and with "a way out" of the crisis, namely treatment. Make no mistake about this: when you create a crisis in the life of an addict, there is always the risk of suicide.

TREATMENT

Group Therapy

"Why do I have to go to group? I wouldn't even speak to these people if I saw them out in public? Besides that, I can afford individual therapy." Charles is an oral surgeon, addicted to nitrous oxide, and mandated to treatment.

This rather obnoxious outburst was delivered in an angry tone on Charles's second day of treatment when a nurse prompted him to go to group. Taken at face value, this might just be a manifestation of a disruptive personality disorder. He might have frontal lobe impairment from his addiction. Then again he might just be an arrogant jackass. Personality aside, his question is legitimate. If I ask you to do something, I should be able to offer you a sound therapeutic reason for doing it.

We are gregarious creatures, and we function naturally in groups, all sorts of groups. We have work groups, church groups, team groups, family groups, friend groups, etc. Living in emotional isolation is difficult and painful. Addiction isolates us from others both internally, due to emotional constriction, and externally, due to our attitudes and behaviors. Recovery in isolation is very difficult.

My answer to Charles's question is this. In my clinical experience, if your addiction has progressed to the point of needing formalized care, not only is some form of group process appropriate, it is also essential. You are out of touch socially, psychologically, and spiritually. You need help to make it back to reality.

By the way, I do not automatically interpret not wanting to go to group as resistance to treatment. It might be simple oppositional behavior or it might be something else. Therapeutic groups can induce apprehension, especially if you have social anxiety or social phobia. For that matter, groups in general may be scary for you.

With that in mind, here is a short version of why we promote group therapy for the treatment of the addicted person and why we think it is so important.

The group process offers positive reinforcement among peers. The shared common denominator or goal of a treatment group is that members want to free themselves of their addictions. It is people helping people within the guidelines of a therapeutic process. It is a process that offers acceptance, understanding, support, feedback, encouragement, self-confidence building, problem solving, purpose, and community. Group offers the addict a powerful recovery opportunity, but it only works if you work within it. As my sponsor said to me, "You won't recover sitting in the back of the room with your arms folded."

Groups provide positive peer support and encouragement. It is inspiring to see others recover and overcome obstacles. Interaction between group members within a professionally led, structured environment actually reduces anxiety and helps with the development of healthy coping skills. Group participation is rewarding and decreases the tendency some addicts have to isolate. Some addicts are initially avoidant of any group process due to social anxiety. These same people tell me later that the group process actually helped lessen that curse.

"I'm Wayne and I'm a drug addict. Wow! I never thought I could sit in a room full of people and say that. Actually, I never thought I could even walk into a room full of people, at least not without being loaded up on dope. I have always had this fear of

groups. Even as a kid I felt out of place. And as for speaking in public, forget that! Now here I am chairing an AA meeting. It still does not seem real at times. I admit it was rough at first. I just sat there in meetings and tried to be invisible. Then, I started talking to people after the meetings and then I got up the courage to introduce myself instead of saying 'I pass.' Nobody made fun of me. You all accepted me and did not judge me or push me. I am saying all this now because I just want to be able to help others like me. I am not cured by any means, but at least I do not have to avoid the big family Thanksgiving this year. And I do not have to get loaded for it either. Thanks guys." Wayne is twenty-two years old. His initial diagnosis was marijuana dependency and social phobia. He's been sober seven months.

There are many different types of group therapy. For our purposes, we will touch upon the more established types used in addiction treatment.

Psycho-educational Groups are facilitated by a leader to provide interactive education, relating to the disease of addiction. Topics include facts about the biological, psychological, social, and spiritual consequences of addiction. These usually encompass discussions on the disease process, the recovery process, drug effects, medications, nutrition, and the like. There is one important caveat worth stressing about psycho-educational groups. That caveat, or stipulation, is that these groups require a leader who can employ a variety of teaching styles in an atmosphere of mutual respect. Since up to twenty percent of people with addictions have attention problems such as Attention Deficit Disorder (ADD) or Attention Deficit Hyperactivity Disorder (ADHD) the teaching style must adapt to this reality. People with ADD or ADHD may have anxiety and resistance to a rigid type of educational group simply because of past, bad experiences of trying to learn in traditional classroom settings.

Another type of group is a **Skills Development Group** which offers you opportunity to develop and practice skills that will help your recovery continue even in high risk situations like this one.

It is the Christmas Season. You have been out of treatment three months and things are going pretty well. You are getting a handle on your anxiety disorder and have not craved alcohol or Xanax since you entered the program. Your boss, a traditional woman, expects everyone to show up at the Annual Christmas Party. Since you are no fool, you are there with your "better half," who has drifted away to chat with friends probably because of the little tiff the two of you had on the way to the party. There is an open bar and the liquor is flowing. However, unlike, last year's party, you plan to remember this one. You do, however, find yourself getting a little anxious, especially since Barney is the third person to offer you a glass of your favorite bourbon, and it smells really good to you.

"No thanks, Barney, not for me."

"Oh yeah, I forgot, you - uh – stopped – uh - drinking. Sorry."

"It's OK. I'm good."

"Heh! Wait a minute." Barney searches through his sports coat and produces a pill bottle half full of Xanax. He shoves them into your hand and says, "Merry Christmas!" as he staggers off.

Do you have the skills to get through this? Do you

have the motivation to get through this? Will you get through this?

Skills Development Groups in addiction treatment focus on recovery skills. Group goals include learning "refusal methods" and how to successfully handle high risk situations like the one in the above scenario. Through a process called "role playing," you can actually rehearse this or similar scenarios in the group process. You get not only the benefit of practice, but also receive input from others on how to successfully handle the situation. The time and place to learn a sobriety survival skill is in the group meeting, not standing alone, in front of a free bar, anxious and angry, with a bottle of Xanax in your hand.

Another recovery technique that is going to come in handy when faced with an opportunity to use involves Cognitive Behavioral Therapy or CBT.

Cognitive Behavioral Therapy is based upon the connections we have between thoughts, feelings, and behaviors. CBT teaches us that behaviors do not just happen. There is a cascade of events that prompts us to act or not act when faced with a situation. The way we act is based upon our **assessment of the situation** at hand. That assessment is based upon our **beliefs**. CBT focuses on eliminating pathological behaviors (like using drugs) by letting us "fix" the unhealthy beliefs (like I can have just one drink) that lead to pathological behavior (like relapse). We can get a brief glimpse into CBT now, but space does not allow an adequate analysis of the process.

Let me tell you how I came to embrace this type of therapy. When I first got out of treatment, I was reading every self-help book I could find because the only education I got about addiction in medical school was how to get amphetamines from the pharmaceutical representatives who hung out next to the elevator by the doctor's lounge. Anyway, I stumbled across a type of CBT dubbed Rational Emotive Behavioral Therapy or REBT in 1979, and I loved it.

REBT was developed by Dr. Albert Ellis. According to Ellis, our interpretation of events is what causes much of our emotional response. Therefore an irrational belief leads to irrational emotions which lead to irrational behaviors.

It goes sort of like this: First there is an **event** in our environment such as a person, place, or thing that triggers an assessment of the situation. Then based upon our **beliefs,** there is an **emotion,** and then there is a **behavior.** We can have a look at this through Jennifer's eyes.

> *Jennifer has been dating this new guy for about four weeks. Even though things are going sort of fast, she is starting to believe this relationship has great potential. This guy seems to be giving out the same signals. One day, she is wandering through the mall and sees him sitting at a coffee shop with a very attractive woman. Jennifer is usually not one to spy, but she stops a moment to take it all in. The two are laughing and sitting next to each other. The attractive woman looks at her watch, gets up, kisses the guy on the cheek, and dashes off.*

> *Jennifer can feel her face flush and her heart rate going up a little. The green monster (jealousy) is creeping up on her. She is starting to wonder if she is being betrayed or played for a fool, and she is getting a little angry. She speed dials her best friend, and they decide she should demand an explanation. He is still sitting there sipping his coffee when she struts up and voices her surprise at seeing him here, especially since she thought he was at work today.*

He stands up, smiles, and tells her that she just missed meeting his sister, but he wants Jennifer to meet her tonight at dinner.

Jennifer is suddenly no longer angry or jealous, quite the opposite, she is gratified. Instead of telling the guy off like she had planned to do one minute ago, she kisses him on the cheek.

The point here is that the event - guy sitting with another girl - was the same event. The difference is Jennifer's interpretation or belief relating to the event. Her first belief was "he is cheating" which induces anger. Her second belief was "he wants me to meet his family," and this induces feelings of gratification. These are normal responses based upon beliefs about the event. She was flexible enough to accept new information and come to a different conclusion which, in turn, produced a different, appropriate emotion and subsequently a fitting behavior or response.

However, what if Jennifer is unable to properly assess the event due to some internal distortion? What if her belief system is so "rigid" and "automatic" that she can accept only one explanation? What if she can only believe that "he is cheating"?

Based upon that rigid belief, let us extend the scenario out for a few more minutes. When the guy tries to explain he wanted Jennifer to meet his family, Jennifer makes a scene and calls the guy a cheating, lying bastard. The guy will probably not consider such behavior an endearing trait. Jennifer will not fare well during the short time remaining in this relationship or in any other for that matter. Her rigid belief system will doom healthy relationships and lead her into pathological ones.

Such rigid, automatic, and self-destructive beliefs are hallmarks of addiction. In its simplest form, the addict sees a drug. The addict rigidly believes taking the drug will cause pleasure and discounts information to the contrary such as repeated adverse consequences. The emotion is excitement due to anticipation of feeling good. The behavior is to take the drug.

Some of the dynamics that perpetuate ongoing addictive and self-destructive behaviors lie within a dysfunctional belief system. In order to correct pathological beliefs one must first identify the problematic beliefs. This entails taking an honest and thorough look into self. Group feedback can assist in identification of maladaptive beliefs. This is an active process, so expect homework outside of group.

Here is an example of a possible homework assignment format:

> **A** - What was the event that resulted in your use of drugs this time?
> **B** - What did you think or believe was going to happen?
> **C** - What emotion did you have?
> **D** - What did you do?
> **E** - What was the consequence?

Here is an example of the assignment as filled out by Rhonda:

> *A - **My activating event** was that my boyfriend scored some heroin. I mean, there it was right in front of me and he asked me if I wanted to use with him.*
>
> *B - **I really believed** I could not refuse. It was overwhelming. I figured I could just use one time.*
>
> *C - **My primary emotion** was excitement. I admit it. I wanted it. I was craving it. I knew it would make me high.*

I was excited.

D – My action *was that I used.*

E – My consequences *were that I could not stop after the first hit. Here I am back in detox, and my parents are talking about getting custody of my daughter from me. Am I just stupid or hopeless or what?*

The "beliefs" that Rhonda needs to challenge in this case might seem obvious but addicts do not change beliefs overnight. Addictive drugs act on the parts of the brain that instill pathological beliefs. The emotional parts of Rhonda's brain actually believe she needs drugs to survive. Her overwhelming goal-directed compulsion is to use drugs. These are automatic ingrained thought processes, and she must develop some competing thoughts and skills to counteract them. We can take a look at her particular irrational thoughts and do a quick analysis of them.

"I could not refuse." This is irrational. Of course she can refuse. There may have been pressure to use, but there was not demand to do so. Admittedly, it would be hard to refuse but not impossible. Irrational thoughts often include "absolute" words like: "should," "always," "never," "could not," and the like. These are words that denote powerlessness.

"I figured I could use just one time." This is irrational. The best predictor of present and future behavior is past behavior. Her past behavior is that one "hit" leads to full blown relapse. She is not playing the whole consequence tape through. She needs to carry the thought process through from taking one hit to losing custody of her daughter.

Her "re-framed" belief about the event needs to be something like this, "If I use, I will immediately get right back into my addiction with all the lying and stealing and legal problems. I will lose my child and alienate my family and I will have no self-respect or self-worth."

With this re-framing, she has a much better chance to refuse using and get the hell away from the person, places, and things calling her back into active addiction.

CBT helps the addicted brain "reframe" thoughts and develop healthy processes and brain circuits, or as an eighteen-year-old addict once told me, *It helps me not think stupid.*

Psychodynamic Groups are led by professional therapists and focus on interpersonal relationships and intrapsychic dynamics. In non-psychiatric language, this is commonly referred to as "getting inside your head" or "finding out what makes you tick." Some people refer to the process as "insight-oriented" group therapy. Labels aside, these groups are based upon several basic concepts.

- Earlier experience affects later experience.
- Perceptions may distort reality.
- You might not be aware of what is influencing you.
- Your behaviors are adaptive and protective in nature even though these behaviors may be self-destructive.

All this makes sense when you are dealing with a brain that has been altered by addictions. Earlier experiences with mood-altering drugs will impact how these drugs effect later and/or ongoing drug use. In short, the earlier you start using, the worse off you are. Drugs distort reality, induce false emotions, and cause pathological learning. The addicted brain actually comes to rely upon drug use and thinks of drug intake as an adaptive or even survivalist behavior. (Example: "It's been a rough day, I need a drink.")

Defenses Encountered in Group Setting: We all have and need psychological defenses. Unfortunately, defenses can become pathological and then instead of protecting us, they can harm us. Things like humor, anger, being a rescuer, being a co-therapist, reverting to a childlike state, blaming, intellectualizing, and rationalizing can work to "protect" our addictions and keep us sick. This is one of the reasons addicts need group therapy. Other group members can see in us what we cannot or will not see in ourselves, and we can see ourselves in others.

Most of these defense mechanisms speak for themselves with the possible exception of "rescuing." It might be helpful to take a closer look at that seemingly altruistic behavior. To do so, we will join in on a group process in action. The counselor has just confronted Sammy about his infidelities in his marriage.

> Sammy: "Yeah. I know I need to break it off with my girlfriend, but there is no way I'm telling my wife about her. My wife has already been on to me about having a girlfriend, and I've been lying about it for years. My wife says I was distant and she tried to fix it. But I just wanted what I wanted. My wife wouldn't drink or drug with me, and my girlfriend would. My wife would criticize me, but my girlfriend accepted me. I love my wife. So I'll just break it off and that will be that."

> Counselor: "So, you're going to let your wife think *she* was doing something wrong all those years and she was crazy? You can't build on a lie, Sammy."

Vern (group member and rescuer): "I agree with Sammy. I think it's best for her not to know. The book says to make amends unless it would harm someone, and that information would harm her."

We can pause the tape right here and examine what just happened. Vern is obviously coming to Sammy's rescue. It would be nice to know what Vern's motivation is for challenging the therapist on an issue that does not appear to impact him directly. Well, it so happens that Vern has a similar secret, and he would rather deflect the conversation away from the topic. He definitely would prefer not to face the music of his wife's knowing about his own affair. Vern is seeking permission to be less than honest. He is seeking permission to relapse. Vern is not rescuing Sammy; he is sabotaging Sammy's recovery. By the way, Sammy's wife has already told the counselor she knows about Sammy's affair and actually "talked" to the girlfriend about it yesterday. She is waiting for Sammy to "get honest or get out."

Groups Based Upon the Twelve-Step Model: These therapy groups are led by a trained counselor and utilize the twelve steps as a model for recovery. Members often receive assignments related to those steps, and successful completion of one assignment is often required prior to moving on to the next assignment or step. This is not an Alcoholics Anonymous peer support group. This is therapy based on the AA model.

There are twelve-step groups that use a modified version of the original twelve steps to fit the addiction and/or the persons involved in the groups.

Again, I want to stress that group therapy based on a twelve-step model is not AA.

Peer Support Groups: These exist, by definition, to provide support rather than give unsolicited advice or confrontation. Peer support groups are widespread and limited to a specific and mutual goal such as staying sober. They are usually focused on sharing experiences and offering pragmatic solutions to challenges one may encounter along the road to recovery. These are often referred to as peer process groups. Participation is ostensibly voluntary, although as I say this, I realize that a judge may order people to attend such meetings as part of their sentence for drug-related offenses such as driving while intoxicated.

These are peer-led meetings and while they may be therapeutic, they are not therapy per se. Examples of addiction related self-help groups based on the 12 steps include:

- Alcoholics Anonymous
- Narcotic Anonymous
- Cocaine Anonymous
- Gambler's Anonymous
- Al-Anon
- CoDA (Co-Dependents Anonymous)
- And many others

Celebrate Recovery is a twelve step program based on eight principles and one Higher Power Jesus Christ).

SMART (Self-Management and Recovery Training) is a peer support group that holds itself out to be secular (non-religious) and scientifically based.

What type of group works best? Actually, they all do. In treatment, there is usually an overlap of the various group techniques. The art is matching the people in the group to the type of therapy that is most beneficial to them. As such, at times, "specialty" groups are the best choices. Some of these specialty groups can be additions to "regular" therapy.

In the following sections, we will limit ourselves to four of these special needs areas and special groups.

Adolescents who use alcohol and/or other drugs are a unique population, and they tend not to mix well with programs aimed at treating adult addicts. Any use of a mood-altering substance is an extremely risky behavior for a person with a developing brain.

Female addicts also have unique needs and issues. Therapeutic interventions that work for males may not work well for females. Female addicted brains differ from male addicted brains. There are distinct biological, neurobiological, psychological, and social issues related to females suffering from addictions.

Male addicts also have unique needs and issues which, if nor specifically addressed, increase the risk for relapse.

Healthcare professionals, both male and female, recover best when involved in specific "cohort" groups in addition to other standard groups and treatment processes.

Our discussion will start with adolescents.

ADOLESCENT TREATMENT CONSIDERATIONS

There are many reasons and variables as to why adolescents use alcohol and other drugs. Identifying these reasons and variables is important so that we as parents and as a society can decrease the risk of our children developing the brain disease called addiction. Here are some factors:

Adolescent Curiosity – This time of rapid brain development is associated with curiosity. It is normal to be curious about drugs and alcohol.

Adolescent Awareness – Since adolescents aware that all types of drugs exist, they need to have accurate information about drugs and alcohol. Adolescents know who the users are in their schools, and they know who can get what. It's no big secret. They are also exposed to the glorification of alcohol via commercial advertising campaigns and other outlets. Adolescents are acutely attuned to their parents' attitudes about alcohol. If a parent uses alcohol in the home, adolescents tend to copy the behaviors of their parents later in life. If the parents disapprove of adolescent drinking, their children are three times less likely to drink alcohol.

There needs to be open and specific communication about alcohol and other drugs within the family. Family values and attitudes need to be discussed. Rules and consequences need specificity in this area. Just to give you an idea of how important this is and how influential parent attitude is for adolescents let us look at a report from the Louisiana Office of Public Health (Volume 22/3 if you want to check it out). "The prevalence (of alcohol use) was sixty-six percent among adolescents whose parents did not feel it was wrong for them to drink alcohol versus twenty-two percent if parents felt it was wrong for them to drink alcohol." Wow!

Adolescent Assessment of Risk – It is not true that all adolescents think they are bulletproof. It is true, however, that if adolescents realize that the downside of use is greater that the upside of use, they will generally opt not to use. Of course, their risk assessment is based upon the information they have to formulate risk. This is an area in which factual and unbiased information can facilitate making an informed decision to use or not use. This is a critical area where parents, family, and teachers can make a real difference.

You will not be present when one of your kid's friends offers him or her drugs. Therefore, it is imperative that he or she has good information about the physical, psychological, and social risks of saying "yes" and the skills to say "no".

Availability of the Substance – Obviously, you cannot use alcohol or any other drug it if it is not available. Unfortunately, it is everywhere. It is in the liquor cabinet at the house; it is in the medicine chest; it is in the grandparents' houses; it is in the houses where the adolescent babysitter sits; it is in the schools; and it is on the streets. Some of it (like hallucinogenic mushrooms) is even growing in the wild – appropriately on cow crap.

Acceptability – If an adolescent's peers ostracize him or her due to a behavior, that behavior will cease or go underground. If the peer group endorses the behavior and puts value on it, the behavior will increase in intensity and frequency. You do not need a PhD in developmental psychology to figure this out. My grandmother knew it: "Tell me who you run with, and I will tell you who you are." Interestingly, overall social norms are also very influential in adolescents. For example, involvement in church activities has protective value against early use of mood-altering substances and subsequent progression into addiction.

Risk Factors for Developing the Brain Disease of Addiction

The ability to delay gratification, at twelve years old, may predict later adolescent alcohol/ drug problems. A test performed at the University Of Washington School Of Medicine shows that putting a high premium on receiving a reward right away (rather than waiting for an even greater reward a week later) is associated with greater risk for use of alcohol and drugs.

Here is the deal. In Phase One, researchers recruited several twelve-year-old twins and got them to do a task. Upon completion of the task the twelve year old could get $7 right away or chose to wait for $10 a week later. Then, in Phase Two, the scientists got them back together two years later for a follow up.

Here is what those researchers found out. If at twelve years of age you opted for the immediate seven dollar payout, you were likely to do the same thing again when you were fourteen years old. More importantly was the discovery that, if you had opted for the seven dollar immediate payout at twelve, you had a six percent chance of marijuana use and a nine percent of cigarette use by age fourteen! The twelve year olds who delayed gratification and waited a week to get ten dollars had a two percent chance of marijuana use and a three-and-one-half percent chance of cigarette use by the age of fourteen years old. (You can check this out at **www.drugabuse.gov**; NIDA notes 12/19/11.)

What this means is that if you help your children learn to

delay gratification, you may decrease their risk of alcohol/drug use.

Genetics: This same study produced some interesting observations regarding genetics. Since these scientists were only doing the research with twelve-year-old twins, they came up with the opinion that genetics influenced the decision-making by thirty percent at twelve. By age fourteen, genetics had a fifty percent part in decision-making. This underscores the need for active parenting and teaching children the benefits of delaying gratification, controlling impulsivity, and setting longer term goals.

There is no single gene that causes addiction. It is generally estimated that fifty percent of the risk of becoming an addict is genetic. Environmental factors (nurture) can override the genetic risks.

Children of Alcoholics: A very interesting finding in children of alcoholics (COAs) concerns the development of two brain structures called the **amygdala** and the **hippocampus**. They are actually abnormal in size and function in some COAs compared to people not raised in an alcoholic home.

One of the amygdala's functions relates to our fear response. A normal fear response is essential for survival. For example, if you are not afraid of lions, you might end up on their dinner menu. Similarly, if you do not avoid risky situations, like drinking alcohol at fifteen years old, you may end up with an addicted brain. On the other hand, if you are afraid of everything, you might want to stay locked up in your house for fear of going out, or you may self-medicate as a form of escape. Or you may end up being totally dependent on someone who will "protect you" and tell you what to do.

The hippocampus stores memories, and COAs generally have plenty of bad memories stored up. The COA's amygdala and hippocampus may be so dysfunctional that they are hypersensitive to negative things in the environment. They may be on full alert at all times and may overreact to what they perceive as a threat. That overreaction may show up as anxiety, irrational fear, avoidance, distancing in relationships, and a host of other problems.

These brain developmental problems appear to be related to ongoing or chronic exposure to severe stress of either an emotional and/or physical nature. Alcoholic family dynamics, as a rule, are pretty stressful. (At least mine were.) It is noteworthy that these types of developmental brain-damaging effects are not limited to alcoholic homes. Any ongoing or severe childhood abuse can result in similar mal-development of these brain structures.

Child abuse can have all sorts of long-lasting and far-reaching consequences. While a complete discussion of these consequences is beyond the scope of this publication, there are certain points that are germane to addiction and addiction treatment. Abused children are at increased risk for the development of addictions, and they tend to have poorer treatment outcomes. The effects of child abuse are both neurobiological and psychological. The internal chaos created by abuse can cause a chronic stress response that is like a silent storm. That storm causes ongoing brain damage even after the abuse has stopped. That chaos shows up as depression, inability to form and sustain intimate relationships, anxiety disorders, social phobias, personality disorders, and of course addictions. Unfortunately, some victims of child abuse find that drugs fill that emotional void or emptiness that can plague them. If that is the case, they are almost instant addicts.

"I hate that bastard step-father of mine. He abused me for years. And my gutless mother did not seem to give a damn either. I guess you could say she was pimping me out to that sick bastard. She even told me not to talk to her about it. I hate her too. He stopped when I was about twelve and had a period, but I always lived in fear that he would start up again. I guess the drugs made it bearable for me. I got some marijuana from a guy at school when I was 13 and then later some Roxies (opiates). Those Roxies made me forget all the pain and crap going on at the house. Roxies let me escape. I mean they worked the very first time. Like - BINGO! I felt normal like other people must feel all the time. I moved out at fifteen. My mother did not dare object because I was going to call the cops on them. I have been through lots of boyfriends since then and a couple of girlfriends, but it never seems to work out. A couple of the guys beat me up, but I know how to get my way with men. That is why I get so many tips at the bar I work in. I have been hospitalized on the psych ward for suicide a couple of times. Well, three to be exact. I feel numb most of the time unless I can get high. But even heroin does not work like it used to. Sometimes I cut myself just to be able to feel. They say I am a borderline personality. The medicines they give me do not seem to work. Sleep? Now that is a major problem. I do not like to dream because it is always bad stuff. That is why I take the Xanax sometimes. I really do not want to die. That is why I am here. I came real close a couple of days ago." Terri is a twenty-two year old female with a history of ongoing sexual abuse from ten to twelve years of age. Her mother is a crack addict. Terri is an opioid addict who transferred to treatment from an Intensive Care

Unit after a near fatal overdose.

As you can see, child abuse, whether it be emotional, physical, and/or sexual in nature, impairs brain development. The resultant emotional, cognitive (thinking), and psychological damage is collectively called mental illness. Child neglect, also a form of abuse, has similar effects.

Age at Time of First Use: If we gather up a group of one hundred alcoholics, preferably sober ones, we could do a survey to see how old they were when they started drinking. The result might surprise you. At least half of the people who were diagnosed with alcoholism as adults had their first alcoholic beverage before the age of fifteen. That is impressive. What is even more impressive to me is that they became alcoholic adults even when they did not have an identifiable genetic predisposition. This goes to show that if you screw up those reward circuits by drinking while your brain is developing, you too can learn to be an alcoholic.

"Oh, yeah, me and my cousins used to get beer at those crawfish boils and go out back and get drunk. It's a part of Louisiana culture. Where are you from? Here? Oh yeah, well you know what I mean. We were all about thirteen years old when we did that. We just kept on doing it. I mean we did not drink every day, but when we drank we drank. Nobody seemed to mind. They were drinking that beer, too, you know. I did get in trouble at sixteen when I wrecked my daddy's truck. Boy, I was some drunk and was going up to the store to get more beer. Oh yeah, they would sell it to us because we said we were getting it for the adults. Anyway, I did not drink and drive after that. Well, I did not drink too much and drive after that. We would all go party in high school and there were times we overdid, it and the coach would get on our asses. But we had fun.

Everybody knows I am the party guy. I like to drink, but I guess I need to stop because it looks like I drank up my marriage and now my job." Bradford is a 36-year-old chemical plant worker referred by his Employee Assistance Counselor in a final attempt to save his job of sixteen years.

Half of the alcoholics in our survey sample started drinking before fifteen years. What about the others? Well, let us ask them this way; "How many of you started drinking alcoholic beverages before the age of eighteen years old?" We will discover that ninety out of one hundred alcoholics start drinking before the age of eighteen. Most of the ninety percent started binge drinking in their teens. Heavy Episodic Drinkers (HEDs) can have measurably decreased brain function in the prefrontal lobes (the decision making brain lobes), especially the female HEDs.

Alcohol is not the only drug this holds true for. It is the same story with cigarette tobacco addiction, marijuana addiction, etc. The younger the user is, the more he or she risks developing an addicted brain and a more severely damaged brain. For the record, early and repeated marijuana use in adolescents causes brain damage. That is a scientific fact.

Energy Drinkers: Adolescent energy drink imbibers are more prone to be sensation seekers, alcohol drinkers, and drug users than those who do not use energy drinks.

Parent - Child Relationships: Positive parent-child relationships are protective against the development of substance use disorders in both male and females. Here is a "close to home" example of how powerful this protection can be. Hurricane Rita had a greater adverse impact on some 14-year-old adolescents exposed to that disaster than others. Research shows that post-hurricane negative life events, such as arguments with parents, illness in the family, and money problems, were significant predictors of increased use of marijuana, cigarettes, and alcohol among these young people. The article is definitely worth reading, especially if you live in hurricane-prone areas. ("Impact of Hurricane Rita on Adolescent Substance Use"; Louise A. Rohrbach, Ph.D., et. al.)

Violence: Witnessing domestic violence is another risk factor for developing addictions as is trauma and/or death within a peer group.

Bullying: While you might expect the victim of bullying to have a greater risk for using mood-altering chemicals, you might not realize that the perpetrator of the bullying is also at higher risk for substance abuse and mental illness. Both the bullied and bullier have higher risks for suicide.

Co-existing Mental Illness: ADHD, depression, mood disorders, conduct orders, Post-Traumatic Stress Disorders, and any mental illness predispose an adolescent to the development a substance use disorder. Early detection of mental illness and appropriate treatment can be protective against substance abuse and progression of the mental illness.

Adolescent Treatment and Recovery:
Sometimes we tend to forget that adolescents are not "small adults." For purposes of this discussion, adolescence is defined as age twelve years old through twenty years old. What works for adults will not necessarily work for adolescents. What works for a younger adolescent may not work for an older adolescent. The prescribing of psychotropic medication to adolescents is not the same as for adults. Indeed, there is concern that these types of medicines can alter brain development. Is this a good thing or a bad thing? Does alteration by medication mean fixing dysfunctional circuits or causing some circuits to stay

dysfunctional or to become dysfunctional? The answer is, I do not know.

Every doctor-patient decision must be individualized, and the risks of prescribing medication must be weighed against the benefits. In the case of prescribing for adolescents, it is my opinion that the benefits should greatly outweigh the risks. I believe this because the risks are more significant for a developing brain. Dangerous side effects in adolescents include increased risk of suicidality, aggression, agitation, and/or mania. Interestingly, SSRI type antidepressants appear to have less benefit for adolescents than for adults.

Here is another major consideration for prescribing to adolescents. Some research indicates that the use of SSRI's in the adolescent brain may increase the probability of developing an anxiety disorder in adulthood.

If possible, prior to initiating medication, adolescent patients should be detoxified and stabilized at least for a few weeks. That way the effects of the addictive drugs which they were using can get out of their systems and allow their brains to begin recovering somewhat. We used to call addiction the great masquerader because an addict can present with all sorts of psychiatric symptoms that may clear up once the adolescent cleans up his or her brain. Given the relatively high risks of these medications, other therapeutic interventions may prove more beneficial and lessen or eliminate the need for medications.

If psychotropic/psychiatric medications are indicated and subsequently prescribed, close monitoring by the prescriber and family is warranted. The patient's therapist must be included in this loop. The adolescent needs to be aware of possible adverse effects and instructed on the need to notify someone immediately should side effects occur. Once the medications have reached a steady state in the patient's brain, ongoing monitoring of the symptoms for which the medication was initially prescribed should occur on a regular basis. If maximal benefit is obtained for a period of time, the prescriber may decide to slowly discontinue the medication to evaluate how the patient does without it. This must be done gradually and under the supervision of the prescriber. Again, the patient's therapist needs to be aware of this process.

One major variable in all of this is the level of patient compliance in taking the medication.

Family Therapy heads the list of adolescent treatment needs. Many times the adolescent's addiction has been progressing "under the family's radar." Behaviors that signal drug use may be attributed to "normal adolescent development" or labeled as "just a phase she is going through." There may be other problems within the family that defocus attention from the adolescent's addictive behaviors. Parents may realize there is a problem, but they may also try to fix it by doing the wrong things for the right reasons. The net effect here is that the drug use escalates.

Damaging effects of drugs on the developing brain can cause developmental retardation. Therefore, a young drug user may present with distorted values and morals, emotional retardation, decreased ability to problem solve, decreased ability to establish realistic goals, as well as other thinking impairments. These impairments also weaken the bonding capability of the adolescent toward the family system. This distancing promotes more drug use. It is a vicious, destructive cycle that needs to be interrupted. Bonding with and belonging to family are very powerful influences to the adolescent and often a primary key to positive behavioral change.

Whatever the specific situation, family therapy can establish, support and/or promote effective communication, system healing, effectual parental monitoring, and establishment of boundaries and acceptable behaviors within the framework of the family's values.

Motivational Interviewing and its counterpart Motivational Enhancement Therapy are particularly well suited for adolescent treatment and interface well with CBT which we have reviewed already. Motivational Enhancement Therapy, or MET, avoids confrontational power struggles with adolescents who, as any parent knows, may already be resistant, rebellious, and narcissistic.

A basic tenant of change is that people support what they help create. For instance, I am much more likely to accept and support a concept if it is my idea. MET builds on this characteristic through a non-confrontational process. MET allows the individual to self-motivate into recovery by tapping into her internal motivation for change. The therapist assesses the stage of a person's motivation and begins the process there. The MET therapist is supportive and empathetic and in essence guides the patient into an introspective journey while utilizing suggestions and feedback the purpose of this journey is to allow the person to gain insight into the reality of her pathological relationship with drugs. Once there is an internalization or realization that a problem exists, she can make a decision to seek treatment or keep on using. If her decision is to seek treatment, she is vested in the process, because it's her idea. If that is the case, this person may be appropriate for a less intense level of care.

If the person elects not to embrace any change, treatment per se may be a waste of time, resources, and energy. If this is the case, family members must decide on their own course of action. Some will elect to force the addict into treatment against her wishes.

Putting someone into a treatment setting against her wishes may actually have a positive outcome. Resistance to change may indicate the need for a more structured recovery environment such as that offered in an inpatient setting. Inpatient placement does give the addict a "time out" and allows exposure to the possibility of a better life without alcohol/drug use. It also allows time for both acute and sub acute detoxification and clearing or at least improvement of the thinking process. If the person is exposed to a strong, healthy patient community, the "recovery attitude" might be contagious.

On the other side of that coin, putting a person into a treatment setting against her wishes may serve to increase resistance and ultimately have the adverse effect of making her "treatment wise." A "treatment wise" addict learns to "play the treatment game" in order to placate others but plans to resume the addict lifestyle as soon as the "coast is clear." Sometimes people are just not ready to change, and they have to go back out and receive more consequences. Unfortunately, those consequences may be severe, long-lasting, or even fatal to the addict and/or others.

A **Contingency Agreement/Contract** can help the adolescent strive for a positive outcome. Recovery has got to be rewarding, or it will not happen. The adolescent brain is supposed to be looking for motivators to wire its reward circuits and centers accordingly. That is how the foundation for adulthood is formulated. Those adolescent brains are learning by trial and error. We as adults are supposed to provide some boundaries within which that process takes place. The first boundaries the child experiences are under the aegis of the parents.

In the "recovery world", as is true in the "normal world",

the types of rewarding activities need to exclude drug use and drug lifestyles if the individual is to be successful. We have already talked about how drugs hijack the brain's reward systems and distort goal-directed behaviors. Providing boundaries can guide an adolescent away from drug use and toward healthy brain development.

A useful therapeutic tool in the addiction field is the contingency contract. Contingency contracts are often employed in the treatment of adolescents. It is a written agreement, between parent and child that defines boundaries. The contingency contract is built on the understanding that a positive behavior will be rewarded and a negative behavior will be punished. It actually provides a sort of "real world" experience.

The agreement, replete with identified rewards and punishments, can be negotiated in the presence of a therapist. Rewards and punishments are usually based upon privileges such as staying up until midnight on Friday, getting to use a cell phone, or borrowing the car. Drug screening must be a built-in component. We can review this sample contract that was negotiated by a therapist between Tommy and his parents to get an idea of what such an agreement entails.

> Tommy, fifteen years old, is insistent that he can stop using drugs if he goes to an outpatient program. He is very resistant to any type of residential care. He is so sure that he can do it as an outpatient that he is willing to enter into a formal behavioral contract.
>
> Some of the provisions of this particular contract are:
>
> - I agree to abstain from all mood-altering substances.

- I will submit to random drug screens every week. If there is a positive, I will immediately check into the residential treatment program and stay for the duration of treatment.

- I will attend outpatient faithfully, and any absence must be excused in advance. If I fail to do this, I will immediately check into the residential treatment program and stay for the duration of treatment.

- I agree to bring my grades up by one letter grade next report period, and I get my X-box back when I do.

Tommy is pretty confident about these external controls keeping him straight. *"I know I'll stay clean with this over my head. Plus, if someone wants me to use, I'll tell them I cannot because I'm being drug screened."*

Of course, any contingency contract is only as good as the willingness of the parents to follow through. In this situation they were willing and serious. Tommy and his using buddies figured out that he could binge drink on Friday and produce a negative urine drug screen for alcohol or alcohol metabolites by Monday. This is exactly what he began doing after about six weeks. His parents noted a change in behavior. The addictionologist ordered a special blood test that could tell if the person had binged on alcohol within the past three weeks. Tommy is currently enjoying recovery at a sober living house in Arizona, far away from all his pathological peers.

Therapeutic community (TC) are drug-free residential houses that use a hierarchical model and treatment stages based on increased levels of personal and social responsibility. Positive peer influence is used to help individuals learn and practice effective social skills.

For some young recovering addicts, this is a process of habilitation rather than rehabilitation since they are learning for the first time the behavioral skills, attitudes, and values associated with socialized living.

TCs tend to have their own cultures and personalities; therefore, matching the person to the facility is important. I want to emphasize the need for due diligence prior to making a selection. Knowledgeable therapists and addictionologists in your community generally keep abreast of how healthy various sober houses are via the proverbial and omnipresent grapevine. I strongly encourage checking with them prior to making a choice.

<u>Adolescent AA</u> can help adolescents, who are addicted. They can benefit from mutual support of self-help groups such as AA, NA, SMART, and Celebrate Recovery. However, availability of such groups may be limited. There is a greater likelihood of finding an Adolescent or Young People's Alcohol Anonymous group than finding any of the others. There are several important caveats, however. Adolescents are vulnerable and must be protected from predators. A safe environment that does not tolerate deviant behavior, including but not limited to drug dealing and/or using, must be in place. In my opinion, some type of monitoring process, by responsible adults is essential.
.

In summation, treatment of adolescent substance use

disorders is very complex. These patients require proper assessment, family involvement, a variety of treatment techniques, and an individualized treatment approach. Even with these factors in play, there are no guarantees. The earlier we can intervene and disrupt the active addictive disease process, the greater the chance of harm reduction for the adolescent brain, the adolescent as a whole, the family, and our community.

FEMALE ADDICTS
<u>TREATMENT CONSIDERATIONS</u>

Some treatment programs offer gender-specific groups while others utilize "mixed" groups. There are facilities that are so gender-specific that they only admit one gender in the entire facility. I have treated patients in all of the above. At the time of this writing, I am the consulting addictionologist for an all-male program and the medical director for another facility that is all-female. So the question becomes what is the best option.

The answer, of course, is both of them. There are pros and cons to everything. I think the pros outweigh the cons in favor of gender-specific groups in the early phases of treatment such as inpatient/residential and partial inpatient. Partial Inpatient is also known as a Partial Hospitalization Program or PHP. The patients come to the facility and participate in all inpatient functions but are not housed at the facility. In an Intensive Outpatient Program or IOP, the patients generally come to a facility in the evening for about three hours a day for three-to-four days of the week. By design, a person who qualifies for IOP is not as deep into addiction as a person who requires inpatient or PHP. There are specific guidelines for matching a patient to a level of care. The guidelines, or patient placement criteria, that I utilize are published by the American Society of Addiction Medicine (ASAM).

Offering gender-specific groups in Inpatient and PHP is supported by addiction research and just as importantly by first-hand experience. There are multiple clinical and social considerations that favor gender specific groups. Not the least of which is the fact that the last thing an addict needs, in the acute phase of treatment, is romantic involvement with another patient. That behavior not only sabotages one person's treatment, it sabotages that of both parties. Just for clarity, there is no real romance going on in such a liaison. At best there is mutual lust, but it generally goes pathologically beyond that.

So-called "treatment romances" are also a way to get thrown out of treatment. I have observed situations in which an addict seduces another patient with the intent of getting kicked out. An addict who tends to run from painful issues may entice another patient by whatever means available, in this case sex, in order to avoid dealing with personal issues in therapy. Running or avoidance has its own reward. Every time the addict avoids a painful issue by running from it, there is some relief or a feeling of escaping pain. After a while, running becomes both rewarding and self-destructive, and the addict edges further into the oblivion of addiction. Not only does the avoided issue not go away, it becomes even more threatening to the addict. The fantasy of teaming up with another addict in treatment and escaping together may seem like a solution to the problems at hand to the addicted brain, but I assure you, it is not. That fantasy never plays out as planned and both generally resume using drugs as well as each other. Neither person can be said to be in relapse because neither was ever in recovery.

If you recall, I said earlier that there is ultimately a common pathway involved in the brain disease of addiction. That pathway is via the brain's reward systems. Sex can give a momentary boost to that pathway and, as such, clandestine sexual liaisons during treatment amount to little more than using. Casual sex is just another form of addictive behavior.

Some addicts have told me that they used sex in treatment as "a way to feel wanted" and to bolster low self-worth. In reality, being objectified in this manner tends to have the opposite effect on self-worth. This behavior is also a selfish disregard and disrespect of other patients.

Sexual liaisons in a treatment center can be quite disruptive to the whole patient community because other patients get involved in secret keeping and "signing off" on the behavior by being part of a conspiracy of silence. This can invoke "junkie" or "street" attitudes such as "not being a rat." In addition to that, dysfunctional addict family dynamics can come into play.

Sexual acting out can also be predatory in nature. Some women are especially vulnerable to predation upon entering a treatment center.

Oftentimes, when a woman enters treatment, her marriage is in trouble. She feels unwanted, may fear abandonment, and has an emotional void to fill. The therapist sees her as dangerously vulnerable. The sociopathic male addict may see her as an easy target.

> Katrina, thirty-seven years old, is an opiate and benzodiazepine addict who has been in treatment for three weeks. She is in my office explaining to me and her female therapist why she should not be kicked out of treatment for having sex with another patient by the name of Harold last evening.

> *"My husband has been angry with me since he found out I was buying drugs. He has called me some really bad names and he has threatened to take the children from me. We have not slept together in months. It is my fault. I keep lying to him, and I spend the house money on drugs. He thinks I am screwing every drug dealer in town. He says this treatment is the final straw. If I do not get well, he is divorcing me and getting custody of the kids. He has already talked to a lawyer. I have been trying to do right by him and my kids, but he takes all that for granted. He takes me for granted!"*

"I know none of this is an excuse, but Harold made me feel attractive and smart and funny. He laughed at my jokes and told me how pretty I was and opened doors for me and smiled at me during education groups. I mean here was this young attractive male wanting me. Me! You cannot let my husband know about this. I cannot afford to be kicked out of treatment. I will lose everything. I know I was stupid."

"Wait! Oh, my god! You don't think Harold has a disease or anything, do you? He said he did not. Does he?"

Harold, the above mentioned twenty-four year old, is an attractive heroin addict with narcissistic traits, Hepatitis C infection, and is on Valtrex for genital herpes prophylaxis. He has this to say, *"Look, I am a man. Okay? And that cougar has been throwing it in my face since she got here. I am sorry, but she got the best of me, and I screwed her. I know it is against the rules, but I do not see the big deal. It is just sex."*

This vignette illustrates the value of gender specific groups. There is a normal bonding process that occurs in group therapy. In early recovery, people are vulnerable. That is why there are strict professional-patient boundaries. Gender specific groups allow patients to focus upon themselves and their issues without distractions from the opposite sex. Plus, there are sexual predators in treatment as well as in outside-self-help groups who act out their own pathology at the expense of others.

We also realize that people who have same sex preference are in gender specific groups, and treatment romance must be addressed in those situations, also.

The fact of the matter is that there is a common denominator for both men and women in treatment – addiction. The other facts are that gender differences give support to the practice of providing specific groups for women in recovery.

Co-existing disorders – Many women with addictions have significant trauma and abuse issues with resultant Post Traumatic Stress Disorder. However, not everyone who experiences trauma develops PTSD. I say this because I don't want people getting labeled solely because they were traumatized. Women also tend to have more co-existing disorders including anxiety and depression. Interestingly, women with Restless Leg Syndrome are more likely to experience depression. Women who experience family conflict at the ages of eleven through thirteen have an even greater risk of developing a substance use disorder than their male counterparts.

Female Physiology and Drugs – Females incur greater damage from alcohol consumption. Indeed, alcohol increases the risk of breast cancer in females. Females are more susceptible to cocaine addiction and methamphetamine addiction and have a greater response to drug cues than males. Female cigarette smokers have less success of quitting. Females metabolize Ambien (zolpidem) differently than males, and eight hours after taking it can still be impaired from the drug. A female's risk for going to an Emergency Room due to taking Ambien are over twice that of a male's. Alcohol may disrupt menstrual cycles. Opiates disrupt menstrual cycles. Female physiology makes them more susceptible to the effects of opiates. For example, one thirty mg Roxicodone pill taken by a male is the equivalent of one and one fourth Roxy or 45 mg if taken by a female. This fact is another glaring reason why the severity of addiction cannot by judged simply by the amount of drugs taken. Addiction is about what the drug does to the brain's reward system.

There is also increasing evidence that estrogen may play a greater role in sex-based addiction differences than previously thought. You may wonder why we are just figuring this out. One of the reasons is that most of the early research on alcoholism involved male alcoholics. This makes sense when you realize the easiest place for information to be gathered by governmental sponsored researchers was the Veterans Health System and early on there was not an overabundance of alcoholic females in that system. In short, the early research conclusions and subsequent treatment recommendations for addictions may not wholly apply to female addicts. Fortunately, research on the female addict has come a long way since then and continues to evolve.

Social Factors – Women seem to carry more guilt and shame about their addictions. Even in this age of enlightenment, there is greater social stigma attached to female addicts. This may stem in part from the fact that women are often viewed as caretakers in the home and are tasked with instilling virtue and values in the children. This bias is pervasive in our society and even makes its way into the doctor's office. Which may, in part, explain why a female patient is more likely to get a benzodiazepine prescription from the doctor than a male patient.

Females are often introduced into drug use by males such as boyfriends. It is not uncommon for a woman to be in a relationship with a male who not only takes drugs, but also supplies her with them. A female-male relationship based upon drug addiction can be more dangerous for the female partner. Women, more than men, are the recipients of domestic and sexual assault. In the USA, a woman is assaulted and/or beaten every nine seconds! That means by the time you finish reading this paragraph, two women will have been severely beaten and/or raped.

There is one more gender difference that stands out in my field. Male spouses tend to leave female addicts twice as often as female spouses leave male addicts.

Involvement in Treatment – Women are more likely to engage in group therapy, and they have less relapse risk while actively engaged in treatment. Females tend to relapse due to interpersonal problems and negative feelings. Male addicts, in early recovery, are more likely to relapse when things are going relatively well. It is also noteworthy, that women may feel more pressured to stay at home and therefore not attend mutual support groups as often as their male counterparts.

Then there is the premature husband. (It is not what you think.) This is the guy who comes to a family session or a family visit ostensibly to help his wife who is in treatment. Of course, his not-so-hidden agenda is to have her come home, no matter how prematurely.

> *"Well, I have got to tell you, honey, that we are all proud of you for doing this, and we are all ready for you to come home. Little Sissy (the three-year-old daughter) cries for you every night. I know you were overwhelmed and depressed and that is why you drank and took those pills. I have also been talking to your family, and we think you could finish all this up in that outpatient program your sister went to. But I do not think you're as bad off as she was. We do need to get back to church as a family, and you can get some counseling there if you need it. I figure you realize all the damage and hurt you have caused, and that right there is enough to stop you from using that stuff. If you say you will not use again, that is good enough for me. You are not like these alcoholics and addicts in here.*

You have got a husband and children and a place to live and a family that loves you. We need you back."
"Honey's" husband.

I have witnessed variations of this theme on all too many occasions, and it is pathological at so many levels. The husband is shoveling guilt and shame all over her. His obviously rehearsed diatribe is peppered with veiled (and not so veiled) threats, and he has even enlisted her family into his self-serving mission of sabotage. And the saddest thing about this manipulation is that she usually follows his lead and signs herself out of treatment and back into the dysfunction that got her here in the first place.

You have got to wonder why her husband would in essence pull her out of treatment. We can speculate about all types of reasons. He might be embarrassed that his wife is an alcoholic/addict. There may be an element of global family denial. Which usually means the social and interfamily shame may not be tolerable within the extended family system. He and other family members may just be ignorant. He might have his own secrets that he would rather not come out in a family session. This is especially true of an extramarital affair. He may beat or abuse his wife. He may be totally dependent on her. He may need her home to work. He may want her to relapse so he can get custody of the kids. He may just be a self-serving personality disorder (jackass). Who knows? Then again, maybe it is because he is basically just as sick as she is or even worse off than she is. Whatever the case, I hope they survive the next crisis and get some appropriate help somewhere.

Pregnancy and Addictions – Detoxification

We talked briefly about this earlier, but now we'll go into a little more detail. The rate of use of illicit drugs during pregnancy is at an alarming four-and-one-half percent nationwide. It gets worse; up to twelve percent of women report binge drinking during the first three months of pregnancy, and the pregnant females between fifteen and seventeen years old use even more than the general population. We see the consequences to the babies in the form of birth defects, some of which are subtle and others which are obvious. The early consequences to these innocent children come in the form of decreased fetal growth, decreased brain development into childhood and beyond infant alcohol syndromes, and/or other drug withdrawal syndromes. Understandably, pregnancy impacts treatment decisions at multiple levels. The most dangerous treatment time for mother and fetus is during detoxification. We have discussed the fact that early drug use causes greater damage to the developing person. A fetus is a developing human, and drug use by mom equates to drug use by this developing human.

Detoxification of Mother and Fetus - requires special care and expertise. The effects that detoxification medications might have on fetal developmental are of major concern when choosing the medications to be used during detoxification of a pregnant addict. All detoxification considerations center on minimizing fetal distress. The process is often complicated by the fact that mom may experience significant mood changes during the prepartum (before delivery) as well as postpartum (after delivery) periods of her pregnancy.

Given the association between bipolar disorders and substance use disorders, providers and patient alike must be especially vigilant for exacerbation of bipolar symptoms during pregnancy.

Opiate Withdrawal and Pregnancy - Ongoing heroin addiction during pregnancy is associated with poor outcomes and endangerment to both fetus and mother. The same can be said for the "legal" short-acting opiates like hydrocodone and oxycodone. Some physicians elect to maintain the mother on methadone or buprenorphine through delivery and treat the infant for opiate withdrawal once the child is born. Ostensibly, the main reason for this opiate maintenance therapy option is to decrease the propensity of the mother to use heroin during pregnancy. Obviously, if the mother is getting methadone or buprenorphine, the fetus is getting it also.

That being said, there are pregnant addicts who want to detox during pregnancy, and if they cannot find someone to help them, they may do it on their own. If mom wants to detox, I am 100% supportive of her decision, and therefore, I do a relatively good deal of high-risk pregnancy detoxification.

If mom is an addict, she is bathing the brain of her fetus in opiates. This is a sure way to highly increase the child's risk for later addiction and other neurological problems. I believe that the longer the fetus is exposed to opiates, the more damage his/her brain accrues. The sooner mom stops using, the less exposure there is to the fetus. However, if mom stops abruptly, the stress of fetal withdrawal can cause fetal damage.

When detoxifying pregnant opioid addicts, I prefer to stabilize mother and fetus on buprenorphine first and then gradually taper the dosage. My rationale for this is that I want to limit the exposure of the fetus to opiates, but I do not want to cause undo fetal distress by detoxing them too rapidly. If mom is detoxing, the fetus is also detoxing, and this is distressing to the fetus.

Subsequently, the best course of action is to limit the time the fetus is exposed to opiates including detox medications but not to detox either mom or fetus too quickly.

It may be safer to detox mom and fetus during the second trimester to decrease the risk of spontaneous abortion (miscarriage). There are no sure-fire guarantees as to outcome with either the gradual tapering detox or with opiate maintenance. The mother must be actively involved and adequately informed prior to making the decision with her doctors as to which course of therapy she prefers to take. There are numerous variables; however, either way she must be monitored closely by an obstetrician and addictionologist during her high-risk pregnancy. This includes monitoring of mom with clinical observations and vital signs. It also includes monitoring fetal heart rates and having mom report things such as fetal activity/movement.

Another goal for detoxification during pregnancy is to eliminate the risk of the newborn child having to go through opiate withdrawal. Clearly, if the infant does not have to go through acute opiate withdrawal at birth, he or she is much better off. The infant withdrawal syndrome can last for several weeks and there is an associated risk of Sudden Infant Death Syndrome (SIDS) in these babies.

If mom is using opiates up to the time of delivery, the child will undergo drug withdrawal. This withdrawal in a newborn baby is called the Neonatal Abstinence Syndrome.

The baby usually starts detoxing in about 24 to 48 hours after birth but may not get "drug sick" until a week or two after delivery.

As you would expect the baby's nervous system is rebounding from the drugs and is hyperactive during withdrawal. These babies are very stressed out and irritable. They have "the shakes" and muscle tightness (hypertonia). They tend to cry a lot which is no surprise to anyone who has gone through opiate withdrawal (it hurts). The baby's cry may be described as "high-pitched." Up to one out of every twenty of these poor babies has seizures. They also have trouble sucking and swallowing so they may vomit and suck the milk up into their lungs and get aspiration pneumonia. They also get diarrhea and dehydration. They get the yawning, and sweating just like any other opiate addict.

This withdrawal process lasts for a week to several weeks but the intensity tends to decrease over about 30 days. The post-acute withdraw syndrome (babies get it too) can last about 6 months.

Alcohol Withdrawal and Pregnancy - From my perspective, there is no safe amount of alcohol consumption during pregnancy. Heavy and/or regular intake of alcohol by mom can result in in a wide range of permanent fetal abnormalities known as Fetal Alcohol Spectrum Disorders. Withdrawal from alcohol in a physiologically dependent pregnant woman is a medical emergency and best accomplished in a hospital setting.

Benzodiazepine Withdrawal and Pregnancy -If the pregnant addict presents in a state of acute benzodiazepine withdrawal, hospitalization and stabilization are needed. Benzodiazepine withdrawal can certainly result in fetal distress and even miscarriage. Once mother and fetus are stabilized, it may be appropriate to transfer the patient to an addictive disease treatment center with detoxification capabilities. Since benzodiazepine (BZD) withdrawal may be a relatively lengthy process, detoxification can continue in an addiction treatment facility that has capable, knowledgeable staff, and appropriate obstetrical access. BZD withdrawal can be quite complicated in non-pregnant patients. These complexities can be magnified during pregnancy.

If the mother elects to continue taking BZD during pregnancy, the new-born may manifest a benzodiazepine neonatal withdrawal syndrome. In neonatal withdrawal, the child will exhibit decreased muscle tone (floppy baby), decreased breathing, tremors, problems eating (poor suck reflex), and irritability. These symptoms may persist for days, weeks, or even months. This in turn is going to have an adverse effect on bonding.

Prepartum Mood Changes - Postpartum Mood Changes - Relapse

While many women stop using when they find out they are pregnant, if you are an addict, there is a real grief process associated with giving up your drug of choice.

> *"We are being honest here, right? And this is not going to be used against me anywhere is it? Ok then. Yes, when I got pregnant I needed to stop using everything, and I did, but there are times when I miss taking it (the drug) especially when I am anxious or depressed or just worried. I would never do that to my baby, but I get really down about it sometimes, then I feel even guiltier for even thinking about it."* Karen is a four-month pregnant patient detoxified from Lortab and Xanax.

Karen is telling us that she needs to deal with the grief of giving up her drugs, and she needs to internalize that pregnancy is not just a time to postpone usage. She is also telling us to watch out for symptoms of a mood disorder that may present during her pregnancy. She is telling us that if she does not embrace recovery, she is going to relapse after her child is born.

Once the child has been delivered, there is an increased risk for postpartum depression and for relapse back into addiction. As noted previously, female addicts often have co-existing mood disorders. Postpartum events can worsen these mood problems. The myriad of problems and issues that may arise are beyond the scope of this book. For instance, mother-child bonding can be disrupted by drug relapse and/or postpartum depression, and/or other mood disorder exacerbations.

Suffice it to say, recovery treatment providers should consider these factors and encourage close monitoring during pregnancy and for at least six months to a year after delivery. Consideration should be given to structured living programs for mother and child in high risk individuals. Spouses and other family members need to be educated on what signs to look for in the event mom is getting ill from a mood disorder and/or drug use.

Some states mandate that the pregnant addict be reported to the state's child protection agency. Louisiana does not.

Pregnancy and Addictions – Outcomes

Fetal Effects Due to Alcohol and/or Drugs are one hundred percent avoidable -The adverse effects of alcohol and or drug use by mom can have both temporary and/or permanent effects on fetal development. Mothers who cause such damage to their babies are often fraught with grief and guilt which in turn fuel continued pathological intake of alcohol and/or other drugs. The mother's ongoing addiction then impairs her ability to care for a child that has special needs. A mother's reaction to the realization that she has damaged her child range from total denial and child abandonment to severe enmeshment and overprotectiveness.

If the damaged child suffers from one of the less apparent forms of fetal drug effects, I often see a mother struggling with denial and/or uncertainty. That denial may delay the child gaining access to services that would help him or her achieve full potential.

I have also treated women who did not decide to detox until late in their pregnancies who reported back to me that the delivery went well the baby is "perfect." Unfortunately, that often remains to be seen. Even though the child looks perfect and is a "healthy" baby, neurotoxic substances, such as addictive drugs, when taken during pregnancy, can have long-lasting neurological developmental impact. The brain damage done to these children tends to show up as thinking and/or behavioral problems later in childhood, adolescence, and into adulthood.

It is essential for the child's family to be educated about this potential for damage and to monitor the child's behavior for subtle clues that may indicate a neurodevelopmental problem or disorder. Denial on the part of the mother or other family members may hinder this recognition. Early detection leads to access of appropriate therapeutic assistance early on. It is also imperative that the child's pediatrician have an honest and accurate prenatal history in order for appropriate care to be rendered.

Alcohol and Pregnancy: Alcohol intake during the early months of pregnancy can increase the risk of spontaneous abortion or miscarriage. The fetal effects of drinking during pregnancy are grouped under the title of Fetal Alcohol Spectrum Disorders.

The severe form of FASD is the Fetal Alcohol Syndrome. These children have specific facial abnormalities such as a thin upper lip, minimal development of the groves between the nose and upper lip (smooth philtrum), and smaller eye slits (short palpebral fissures). They are often small in stature.

As expected, since alcohol is a brain-toxic drug, the child with FAS has problems with learning, memory, attentiveness, communication, and/or vision. These children do not do well socially and can easy be targets for bullying.

Another type of FASD is called Alcohol-Related Neurodevelopmental Disorder (ARND). These children can present as learning impaired. They tend to do poorly in school due to decreased cognitive ability. Children with ARND frequently lack attentiveness, and manifest poor impulse control.

FASD children can also exhibit Alcohol-Related Birth Defects (ARBD). Alcohol intake during pregnancy can cause organs other than the brain to be abnormal. These include the kidneys, the heart, the ears, and even the bones.

FASD effects are permanent but early identification of FASD can help caregivers understand the child's needs and offer therapeutic and social support to help the child reach his or her full potential. These children are at high risk for developing alcohol and other drug dependencies themselves.

FASD is one-hundred percent preventable yet two to five percent of school aged children in the United States have some form of FASD. To call this a tragedy is an understatement.

Other Drugs and Pregnancy

Amphetamines: Amphetamine-addicted mothers are at increased risk for pregnancy complications including premature delivery. These addicted mothers are generally using large amounts of amphetamines and methamphetamines far in excess of those legitimately prescribed. People who use amphetamines are often undernourished and subsequently their fetuses are undernourished. Babies born to amphetamine-addicted mothers are at risk for small overall birth size. Larger doses increase the risk for birth defects of the heart. The long-term neurotoxic effects may lead to behavioral problems, attention problems, learning problems, and muscle coordination problems.

Benzodiazepines: Prolonged use, especially in the last three months of pregnancy, can result in an Infant Withdrawal Syndrome which can persist for hours to days to months. Long-term effects of benzodiazepine use by mom during pregnancy may include a predisposition to anxiety and retardation of muscle function development in the child.

Cigarettes: Unbelievably, over sixteen percent of pregnant females smoke cigarettes. This addictive behavior creates risks to mother and child. Smoking during pregnancy doubles the risk of SIDS (Sudden Infant Death) in the baby. Doubles!

Among the myriad of adverse effects on the child is the fact that smoking decreases the blood supply to the fetus, and this is one of the reasons the child may be smaller that he or she should have been.

I ask my patients to think of it like this. Your developing child is getting all his or her nutrients and oxygen thought the placenta. If I told you that I am going to put a clamp on that placenta and squeeze it to cut off the amount of oxygen to your baby, would you agree to that? Of course not! Yet you do that exact thing every time you light up!

Mom's smoking during pregnancy is a curse to the fetus that can result in a lifelong burden for her child that extends throughout adolescence and into adulthood. This curse can result in decreased brain development and a resultant lower IQ than his or her peers whose mothers did not smoke. From a behavioral perspective, children of moms who smoke have more attention problems and more overt conduct problems such as defiant, destructive, deceitful, and/or aggressive behaviors. The brain chemical interference due to mom's cigarette smoking can present as depression and anxiety disorders in early childhood.

When I am doing an intake with a new patient and I get a history of anxiety and or depression during childhood, I ask the patient if he or she knows anything about how his or her pregnancy went. I specifically ask if his or her mother smoked cigarettes during pregnancy. Mom's smoking may have caused disruption of her child's brain enzyme, MAO (monoamine oxidase), and this may point me toward the right medication for her child who is now in his or her twenties.

Regrettably, many of the people I see really do not know much about what transpired when they were in mom's womb.

Cocaine: The "typical" cocaine addict uses the drug intermittently. The adverse effects of cocaine or any other drug on pregnancy are related to multiple factors. These include the time of use during pregnancy, the length of use, and the amount used. Cocaine complications of pregnancy can be very detrimental to both mother and fetus. The fact that cocaine causes blood vessels to powerfully constrict can result in hemorrhages in the placenta and in strokes to the fetal brain. In the fetal brain, cocaine appears to disrupt brain cell development and organization. Long term effects may include subtle brain dysfunction relating to attention and emotional reactions as well as a decrease in development of muscle function.

Marijuana: We have discussed the fact that in order for any mood-altering chemical to alter mood, there must be brain receptors that are activated by the chemical. This means there are natural, internal brain chemicals that act on these receptors. That in turn means the addictive drug is mimicking the natural brain chemicals. For marijuana, the natural substances being mimicked are anandamide and apparently some others.

Anandamide is an endocannabinoid (or internal cannabinoid). It acts at cannabinoid receptors in the brain and the immune system. Marijuana contains the cannabinoid THC as well as other cannabinoids. When a person smokes marijuana, these exogenous cannabinoids (from outside the body) act upon the natural cannabinoid receptors within the body.

When the fetus is fourteen weeks into development, the endocannabinoid system (anandamide) is busy showing nerve cells where to connect with each other. Normal development of these brain circuits can be disrupted by putting external cannabinoids (such as marijuana) into the fetal brain. These disrupted circuits are involved with emotions, learning, sleep, and muscle coordination. Smoking marijuana confuses this developmental process. It is like having too many cooks in the kitchen.

Marijuana is the most commonly illicit drug abused during pregnancy. While maternal marijuana use during pregnancy is not associated with major physical abnormalities, regular use can cause a withdrawal syndrome in the newborn. Regular use also results in long-term effects on brain function. These include anxiety, depression, learning deficits, problem-solving difficulty, memory problems, attention problems, and/or impulsivity problems. There is an association between maternal marijuana use and the development of "juvenile delinquency" in children. This may become most apparent when they become teenagers. These problems tend to persist into adulthood.

Herbal Marijuana Substitutes: Several female patients have asked me about the effects of "synthetic marijuana" on pregnancy. This is a question that is almost impossible to answer. First of all, nobody really knows what synthetic cannabinoids will be in the "synthetic weed" from day to day or batch to batch. The content of this stuff changes without notification. The chemicals are constantly being altered to avoid legal restrictions. There is absolutely no quality control because the stuff is not legal for human consumption. Therefore, nobody really knows all the effects that using synthetic marijuana will have on mom or baby, but preliminary studies indicate there are serious adverse effects.

With so many unknowns, every time someone uses this stuff, they are in essence experimenting on themselves. If you are pregnant, you are experimenting upon that developing human inside you called a fetus. As science catches up with synthetic marijuana, many of these users will be some sort of sad statistic.

There are reports of individual women who have suffered severe pregnancy complications related to this stuff. These compounds cause brain damage in the user, and they cause brain damage with passive exposure to the fetus. Moms who continue to smoke "synthetic weed" during pregnancy will probably give birth to brain-damaged kids. The only question is how severe that damage will be.

Hallucinogens: In determining the effects of hallucinogens on pregnancy, we are confronted with the same problem as with synthetic marijuana substitutes in that we don't know what is in some of this stuff and neither does anyone else including the user. Suffice to say that usage of "hallucinogens" during pregnancy is extremely irresponsible, equates to child abuse, and carries the risk of brain damage to the child.

Opiates: If mom is an addict and her opiate levels are up and down, as they tend to be in addicts, the fetus is getting the same treatment. The fetus is in and out of withdrawal within the womb. As long as mom is actively addicted, this is happening on a constant basis. As previously discussed, if mom delivers the child while on opiates, the child will undergo a withdrawal syndrome called Neonatal Abstinence Syndrome (NAS) which is pretty horrible. Opiates may impair brain cell development and growth. Long term effects include attention developmental problems such as ADHD and behavioral problems.

Polydrug Use and Pregnancy: Most drug users are not purists. They use other drugs in addition to their drug of choice/dependency. Mothers who use drugs during pregnancy are at higher risks for having impaired children. Since about fifty percent of pregnancies are unplanned, a drug-using female is a risk for exposing her child to brain-toxic substances before she even knows she is pregnant.

Not only do the addictive drugs cause fetal brain damage, but maternal stress in and of itself can also have lasting adverse effects on the child. Most active addicts are immersed in stress and chaos which creates a double whammy on the child's brain development. It is imperative that such females get into a recovery process as soon as possible, and they should have priority status for doing so.

Pregnancy and Confessions of a Co-dependent Addictionologist: Sandy is 22 years old, and this is her first pregnancy. She has an infection on her arm due to an IV miss, and I have just told her what antibiotics I am going to prescribe. Her first question is a worthy one: "This won't hurt my baby will it?" I assure her the medications are safe. She leaves my office, goes outside, and lights up a cigarette. Of course, I go out and confront this behavior in the context of motivational interviewing, but I am internally alarmed and outraged by this conduct. Does she not get it? Did I fail to emphasize the effects of cigarettes on her developing child? Does she not understand that she is heaping more damage onto an already at-risk child inside her womb? This is an overwhelmingly powerful disease, and we have to meet the addict where she is and help her work toward recovery. Right now, she is agreeing to cut back and set a quit date. I understand that, and I am going to help her achieve that goal.

I also need to realize that my frustration and feelings are real. I must process them with someone who can understand where I am coming from. I am aware that the doctor who treats himself has a fool for a patient. When I reach out, I am reminded of several treatment axioms. For one thing, I must accept "life on life's terms." Healthcare professionals who care for and treat addicts, especially pregnant ones, must safeguard themselves against negative emotions such as judgmentalism and the like. We (as in me) must also maintain the boundaries of being responsible to the patients and not for the patients. That can get blurry at times and hence the need for a support system. If we do not take care of ourselves and "practice what we preach," we have little to give our patients or anyone else for that matter. At the end of the day, we need to go home knowing we have done "the next right thing" and try not to take it home with us. I am still trying.

MALE ADDICTS
TREATMENT CONSIDERATIONS

Gender influences just about everything including brain development. While there are gross similarities between all human brains, it is blatantly obvious that male brains and female brains differ from each other.

Just as with females, some male behaviors may be "hard wired" into the brain. This is one of the reasons that guys in recovery have their own unique sets of problems. Environmental factors, such as emotional, physical, and/or sexual abuse, also exist for males and have an adverse impact on male brain development. Also, as with females, some problems are rooted in cultural traditions and stereotyping. Even in our equal opportunity, enlightened nation, I frequently encounter young and older men who are anchored in the "manly man" belief systems. Our society challenges those beliefs on the one hand and re-enforces them on the other.

Stereotyping is resistant to change.

Men tend to be more resistant than women about going into therapy. For that matter, men tend to resist going to a health care provider period. "I should be able to handle this on my own" is a mantra I frequently hear from male patients. I hear this when they get into treatment, and I hear this when they blow out of treatment against medical advice. When men do bail out of treatment, the reasons for doing so are not uncommonly veiled behind some male stereotypic smoke screen.

"I am out of here, Doc. All they want to do with that group stuff is break me down and make me cry. What kind of crap therapy is that? I need to know how to stop drinking, not cry about how my daddy

never hugged me. It's like my poor old daddy used to say, God rest his soul, I just need to pull myself up by my bootstraps." Gerald, 33 years old.

Besides bootstraps, Gerald has some other interesting "traditional" beliefs. He is getting progressively more uncomfortable because some of those beliefs are being challenged. Worse than that, the challenges are making some sense to him. This is scary stuff because it threatens his self-concept of who he is supposed to be. His response to fear is like anyone else's. Gerald is ready to fight or flee. Since he is surrounded by all these treatment people, and since "his daddy did not raise a fool," flight is looking like a pretty good option right now.

Gerald believes he should be the breadwinner and head of the household, but he has been laid off and odd jobs are not meeting the financial obligations. He feels like a failure because his wife has to work outside the home. He was okay with her having a job when it was not a necessity, but now it is a necessity. He is very embarrassed about this situation.

Gerald figures actions speak louder than words, so sharing feelings is not something within his comfort zone. He is used to "sucking it up." That is what he was taught to do and that is what he tells his sons to do. Gerald's connection to his wife is very important to him, and he will admit that, but he also admits he rarely tells her that he cares for her. "She knows I love her." The thought of losing her "scares him to death," but the need to be seen as "strong" by her may hinder him from showing it. "A woman wants a strong man she can rely on, and I admit I ain't been that reliable lately, but I have learned my lesson." Gerald figures he can go home and be the man he thinks she wants him to be and just not drink, and everything will work out.

There is one little problem: she will not come pick him up

and is threating a restraining order and a divorce if he does not stay in treatment and sober up. In her words:

> *"I am not going to be like his momma and watch my husband go in and out of jail for drunk driving, act like a jackass, and then die of liver cirrhosis and leave me and the kids to fend for ourselves. I am just not going to have it!"*

If a guy will not stop and ask for directions to the nearest gas station when the orange warning light on the gas gauge is blinking so hard the battery is in danger of dying, what are the chances he is going to spontaneously go bopping up into some counselor's office to talk about intimacy issues? The likelihood of that happening is pretty slim. It is also pretty tragic because men in the USA also commit suicide four times more often than women.

Anger: Anger is a normal emotional response to threats, whether they are real or imagined. Anger promotes aggressive responses. If a dog gets angry, it growls, bares its teeth, and bites. Hopefully, we've come a little further up the chain than our canine buddies, but at times I wonder about that.

Humans tend to express anger in a variety of ways. Acknowledgement of anger and the appropriate expression of that emotion is healthy. Unfortunately, the appropriate expression of any emotion is not necessarily the strongest suit for an addict. In the case of anger, this seems especially true for men.

Men often have more anger management issues than women. There are multiple factors for this. Some men use anger or the threat of getting angry to control others. This, of course, creates a dysfunctional dynamic that promotes resistance by the other parties in the relationship. It also forces them into various dysfunctional survival roles. After all, who wants to be held captive by fear?

> *"We do not dare upset Andre because he might "go off" and get drunk. He says some awful things to me and the kids when he is drunk. He stays in a bad mood then he wonders why the kids never let their friends come over. He has never been violent, but he is just so negative and critical all the time. We are all tired of walking on eggshells. Once the kids are up and grown. I will probably leave him [pause] if I can last that long"*

Anger breeds anger. Children who come up in "angry," unpredictable homes may have anger issues themselves which they in turn take into their own relationships.

I have treated guys who actually enjoy anger and are comfortable with it as their predominant emotion. Our cultural glorification of violence in the entertainment media contributes to this somewhat. The male protagonist or hero is often portrayed as a violent person who is respected and rewarded for his violent behaviors.

For men with anger problems, rage is frequently bubbling right below the surface, and may be triggered by some seemingly small event. This is especially true if the guy is drunk or loaded on drugs.

For instance, taking an ax to the picnic table on the patio because you hit your shin on it for the third time today because you are drunk, is not normal behavior. At least, that is what one of my ex-wives told me. She was right. I had to make amends about that one.

Ironically, even though anger is a normal, adaptive emotion, some men fear their own anger and try to suppress it or at least dampen it with drug intake which often ends up making it worse. Stuffing it down does not work well either.

There are physical problems associated with pathological anger, including heart disease, high blood pressure, tension headaches, diabetes, and accidents.

If you don't deal with your anger, it will deal with you. Anger management is an important part of recovery. Anger management techniques include cognitive behavioral therapy, relaxation techniques, emotion identification and expression, and learning to think before you act.

Sex: On the average, men tend to have greater sex drives. They think about it more, they pursue it more, and for some men sex equates to conquest. However, men also have a need to connect at an emotional level and to have intimate relationships. Men seem to be wired to compete, to be active in sexual pursuit, and to be less verbal about feelings. Indeed, when it comes to jealousy, men are much more jealous about sexual infidelity than emotional infidelity.

Male addicts often have a degree of sexual dysfunction. Or as my counselor used to tell me, "Fifty percent of the male patients in here report some sexual dysfunction, and the other fifty percent lie about it."

I think he was right. At any rate, male sexuality needs to be addressed at some point in addiction treatment.

Male sexual function is also an issue when it comes to medication compliance, especially with antidepressants. There are antidepressants that will not suppress male sexual function. Plus, keep in mind that at times, the medication gets blamed unjustly. If a guy can't function, the first thing he tends to do is blame the medication. Of course, blames it on the cigarettes. If you are a male, and you are experiencing sexual dysfunction, check with your physician before you go treating yourself by stopping medications. As an aside, some of those "on line" sex supplements are really bad news.

Yohimbine can cause high blood pressure, anxiety, agitation, increased heart rate, and gastrointestinal problems. Anxiety and agitation are major relapse triggers. Other "aids" can promote drug craving, heart problems, bleeding, and hypomania.

Male Relapse: Men tend to relapse behind positive events. Obviously, they relapse behind negative events as well.

> *"Things were really going well; I got complacent. I was out with the guys and the Saints won and I celebrated. Once I did that, I did okay with social drinking for a little while, then I got back into the whole alcoholic drinking pattern. I should have never had that first beer."*

Men who are married tend to relapse less. This is really interesting because women who are married tend to relapse more. Why is marriage protective for males? One reason may be that alcoholic men are often married to non-alcoholic women. As such, there will be less chance of getting drunk with their partner or having that first social drink.

A woman married to a heavy drinker is obviously at more risk for relapse. Men tend to divorce women who are heavy drinkers. Subsequently, the divorced woman may find a man who accepts her drinking. It would not be unheard of for such a man to be a heavy drinker himself.

HEALTHCARE PROVIDER SPECIALIZED GROUPS

Just to clear up any misconceptions, I think it is important to state that healthcare provider groups exist not because these particular patients are "special" or better than other people, but because they have unique needs and issues. Being a healthcare provider, whether it be a doctor, a nurse, a dentist, a pharmacist, a psychologist, or a host of other healthcare professionals, is a sacred trust. By definition, if a healthcare provider is addicted, he or she is impaired and in violation of that trust. The impaired health care provider needs to be in a regular setting and in regular groups with everyone else but also needs additional specialized groups. There are certain issues, fears, and concerns that simply will not be expressed in a "mixed" group. Here some examples:

> *"The kid had a ruptured appendix, but I did not know that at the time. I was relying on the Emergency Department doctor to do a good evaluation, but by the time I got there, the kid was septic. I started antibiotics and did the surgery, but he ended up in Intensive Care. He was in there for seven days, and it was touch and go for a while. I admit that I had a couple of drinks that night, and I had alcohol on my breath. I usually do not drink on call but I did that night. Was it my fault? I do not know. Maybe it was. At any rate, I got reported by the nurses. You all know the drill after that. So here I am. The physician health program sent me here because I might have an alcohol problem. My hospital privileges might be up for grabs. I am not sure what the medical board is going to do. I may end up in the data bank. There is a malpractice suit being filed, and I damn sure do not want them to know that I am in a treatment center. I could lose everything."* Paul, general surgeon, twelve

years in private practice.

"The nursing board sent me here to treatment. I have a problem with Ambien. What happened was that I hung the wrong blood on a patient. She had a horrible reaction. I feel so guilty. I have always considered myself to be a good nurse. I never had any performance problems before, and I got great reviews. I knew I shouldn't be taking that stuff, but it got to be a compulsion for me. I know I did wrong. The sad thing is that I do not even remember doing it." Millie, 37-year-old med-surg nurse.

"I think the stress just finally got to me. You know how it is in the emergency room. We had two codes that night. We did our best, but neither person made it. We all know how hard it is to tell the family someone has just died. Someone they love. I went home that night, and instead of taking my usual 1 mg of Xanax, I took the whole bottle. I ended up in the psych ward, and now I am here. I know Xanax and wine do not mix, but I had been mixing them for over a year before I OD'd." Ray, Emergency Physician.

"I have migraine headaches, or at least that is what I thought. Anyway, I decided to give myself an injection of Demerol one night. Then I did it the next night and the next and the next. I got to where I was using it just to function. Demerol gave me energy. It also got me arrested. I am sure I was probably impaired, but I really did not realize it. I am an addict. I hate to admit it. I am ashamed of it. But it is true. I let everybody down. I thought about suicide but I figured what the hell. I'll give treatment a try. I can always kill myself later if it doesn't work." Me.

Addiction is an equal opportunity disease. If healthcare professionals do not have equal access to treatment, a conspiracy of silence can develop. That conspiracy essentially forces healthcare providers to go "underground." The end result is that healthcare professionals generally do not seek treatment, and they do not report their impaired colleagues. Most impaired healthcare professionals do not seek voluntary treatment for fear of loss of licensure. The impaired healthcare professional continues to suffer, the disease continues to escalate, and patients are at risk. It is a lose-lose scenario. Unfortunately, this scenario is not far-fetched. Indeed, prior to implementation of impaired physician programs in the late1970s, this is exactly what was happening.

Healthcare professionals do require some specialized groups. They also require close monitoring for an extended period of time after initial treatment. Most healthcare recovery contracts require a minimum term of five years. Relapses require immediate cessation of practice.

Healthcare professionals are in "safety sensitive" jobs. They are in a position of public trust. They have easy access to all sorts of addictive medications. Many have a hard time being patients. Many are caretakers who do not take care of themselves or let others care for them. If they are impaired, their patients can be in immediate danger. Plus, healthcare providers tend to under report problems and usage of alcohol and/or drugs. This of course increases the risk that the healthcare addict will be under diagnosed. They often have enablers who protect them.

When confronted or when anticipating "getting caught," they often seek out other colleagues to treat or evaluate them.

"I knew I was going to get reported. I should never have called that patient a fat, selfish, ugly, ungrateful bitch, at least not in front of the nurse but I was pretty amped up on Adderall. And she was being a bitch. So I called up my brother-in-law who is a psychiatrist and went to see him the next day. I figured that would suffice. But the hospital wanted a more thorough assessment, and the board let me know that they frowned upon my self-prescribing. I ended up in treatment. I admit I was overdoing it on the Adderall, but we were short a doctor, and we all had to pull extra shifts. They say I'm a disruptive physician and an amphetamine addict. Am I disruptive because I said what everyone else was thinking? I think not. We've all been there, right?" Gerard, hospital internist, introducing himself to the group.

The healthcare provider seeking treatment and the patients who will be impacted deserve and require the type of treatment that offers the best chance at recovery.

Heathcare providers often require more intense and longer treatment and involvement in what is termed "cohort-specific" groups. The recovery rates for healthcare providers who receive adequate care and follow up in professional health programs is right at 90% over a five-year period.

Licensing boards exist to protect the public (patients). Healthcare professional programs exist to protect the public (patients) and to advocate for the healthcare professional advocacy is not enabling.

Most healthcare professionals who become addicted are loners in their usage. They are very good at concealing their alcohol and drug use. Many are perfectionistic and excel at healthcare delivery until they become impaired. They often have many enablers who make excuses for them or even cover up for them. They often have intense guilt about their behaviors and a great deal of shame that must be dealt with as they re-enter the professional workplace.

Healthcare specific aftercare can assist in the re-entry process and in ongoing sobriety.

THE FAMILY DISEASE OF ADDICTION

Families seek balance or homeostasis. Balance and cohesiveness are maintained in part by "family rules" that reflect family values. Acceptable behaviors are defined and rewarded. Unacceptable behaviors are punished. The values are taught via consistent and clear communication and by role modeling. There is no official rule book per se, and that's a good thing because families also require flexibility. Respect, trust, love, forgiveness, acceptance, and accountability are necessary components. Nobody has the perfect family. We all make mistakes.

Family therapy represents a specialty in and of itself. I am not a family therapist, but I know good therapy when I see it, and I know that family therapy is an integral part of the recovery process. I believe this so fervently, that it is a deal breaker for me. If a treatment program does not have an accessible family therapy component, I do not refer to them. Most treatment programs do encourage family involvement. However, it is not always easy to get family members involved.

Family members may not want to be involved for a variety of reasons. There are family members who tell me that they are "just worn out" and not interested in more therapy centered on a relapsing addict. They have in essence compartmentalized the addict as a toxic influence who is no longer welcome in the home.

> "I finally came to the realization that no matter what I did, I could not control him and that one day I would get the call that he was dead. Once I accepted that, I came to a sort of peace with it. I started to live my own life. I'm ready to help but I am not going to let his addiction destroy me and the rest of the family." This was the response by a wife when asked to be

involved in treatment number four for her estranged husband."

It is also no surprise that some addicts come into treatment to get their families "off their backs" or to manipulate a spouse into accepting them back again. Some addicts even make the treatment center part of their disease process. They do this by using "swinging door" detoxifications. When things "get out of hand" and they end up on the street, they run to a detox facility to rescue them. These frequent flyers are not admitting themselves to get sober but to have a safe place to stay between episodes of using alcohol and or other drugs. They have simply burned up family enabling resources and have incorporated the detox facility into their using cycle and are casting the treatment staff into roles of being enablers.

Some family members resist involvement in treatment because of their own addictions or secrets. Addiction can be multigenerational. It can also skip generations and even appear for the first time in an individual family member.

All sorts of dynamics and liaisons develop within a family system when a member suffers from addiction. Addicts rarely suffer alone. Families protect the family unit, and therefore, members protect each other. Family cohesion is challenged when a member has an addictive brain disease. The addict member tends to exhibit behaviors that violate family values and traditions. He or she generally becomes more and more unreliable as the drug becomes the most important motivator in his or her life. As noted before, other members may try to intervene by doing many wrong things for the right reasons. The following are examples of "wrong" intervention.

> **Enabling:** *"I'm not just going to throw him out on the street. What if he gets killed? I could never live*

with myself. Yes, I give him money, and yes, I even lie to my husband and the other kids, but he is a good boy and he is trying to quit." Mom talking about her addict son.

Bribing: *"Listen, honey, if you just stay here in this program and finish, I will buy you that new Camaro you want and pay your tuition for as long as you stay sober."* Dad talking to his addict daughter.

Rescuing: *"I should have let him sit in jail just to teach him a lesson, but I could not do that. Despite our differences, he is my dad. This is DUI number three. I am working on a deal to get the charges dropped."* Thirty-year-old son talking about his dad who was arrested after a motor vehicle crash in which his mother was injured.

Guilt: *"I blame myself. His childhood was really bad. I was married to a mean alcoholic. If it was not for me he would not be in this situation. I will do anything I can to fix him."* Mother talking about her addict son.

Rationalizing: *"My son did not make it in those other treatment centers because they had unprofessional counselors and a bad program. All he needs is a good program."* Attorney father demanding treatment center number six admit his unmotivated son.

Minimizing: *"Wanda uses a little marijuana, but the judge is overreacting. Her problem is definitely not as bad as the other people in here."* Grandmother who has custody of this adolescent addict.

Living with an active addict's irrationality is like living in an imperfect storm. The addict is in the eye of the hurricane, and the chaos is spinning around him or her. The family energy is focused on trying to manage the unmanageable, and family cohesion tends to suffer as family members are split as to how to address the problem.

> **Splitting:** *"I am sick of my wife lying for my oldest son all the time and going behind my back to give him money. I say kick his ass to the door if he wants to steal from us and run the streets and use drugs. I damn sure do not want him around his younger brother."*

> **Exiting:** *"I am joining the Army as soon as I am of age and getting the hell out of this craziness. I kind of hate to leave my sister in this mess **(survivor guilt),** but she has a plan too. She is going to marry her boyfriend as soon as he gets out of high school and get out. I hope she does not do anything stupid like get pregnant in the meantime. "* David 17 years old.

Even after one escapes from an addict family, they may benefit from therapy aimed at resolving the trauma and beliefs created by being immersed in a sick family system. There is a large knowledge base about children of addicts or COAs.

The problem about running from something is that you may end up constantly reacting to that negative which can lead you right back to whatever you were running from.

> *"I swore I would never be like my mother. I remember her being passed out on the couch surrounded by empty wine bottles, but here I am, a mirror image replete with Xanax, red wine, and two daughters who swear they will never be like me."*

Sara upon entering detox.

Reactive living is little more than survival. Proactive living sets you free.

I categorize the COA phenomenon as a prolonged adjustment disorder in which you learned survival skills that got you through the chaos, but now those same skills are maladaptive and disadvantageous. Some people are affected more than others.

If insanity and chaos are your norms, you may seek the same for yourself. How do you do that? Easy! Marry an active addict, especially one with a borderline personality disorder, and you will be right at home again.

If you are used to inconsistency, cover-ups, and lies, you may be comfortably uncomfortable in such a marriage. If so, you will lie to protect the feelings of your addict spouse. Then you will worry about being a liar. Then you will assume your partner is also a liar but does so to protect you. "He would keep the truth from me if he thought it would hurt my feelings." In turn, you are always seeking reassurance and the chaos and craziness goes on and on and on. Then when things seem as crazy as your family of origin, from which you thought you had escaped, the two of you have a child. Wow!

> *"I was born into a dual-addicted parent home, and my hypervigilance was centered around always waiting for the other shoe to drop. One of the unspoken rules was, "Do not get too hopeful or happy because the crap is coming and it is headed straight for the proverbial fan,* and guess who is standing right in front of it?" ACOA.

This type of belief can readily lead to self-sabotage. It also constricts positive feelings because you are afraid to feel good in expectation that bad feelings follow good ones.

My grandmother once said of her youngest daughter, "She is loyal to a fault." What she was referring to was my aunt's third or fourth husband (I lost count) who was a philanderer. It was not until years later (when I got sober) that I really realized what this meant. My aunt had bonded to this guy and would defend him and stay loyal to him no matter what. That pathological phenomenon would be called "traumatic bonding" today. The deal was that she had abdicated all power to this abusive guy who was "not all bad" and could be "so caring at times." Ironically, she learned it from my grandmother's own relationship with her husband.

Undeserved loyalty can also be anchored in the fear of rejection. Then there is the whole "people pleaser" thing where you do for others to the exclusion of your own needs so people will like you. Alcoholics need caretakers. The result of having one and/or being one is not uncommonly the development of a hostile dependency on the part of one or both parties.

Some people respond to chaotic families by becoming mentally and emotionally rigid. They need to know the rules and everyone needs to play by them. In the search for order, they may exhibit obsessive compulsive traits in which there is a "right time and a right place for everything" and if anything is not in the right place, the person experiences anxiety.

Volumes are written about the dynamics and sequelae of being brought up in an alcoholic or addict household. I have barely scrapped the surface here. If you are interested in child of alcoholic and/or co-dependency literature, there is a plethora of it out there. The book stores are full of volumes upon volumes about it all. Indeed, there are usually so many

COAs and Co-deps cluttering up the self-help book aisle that we could hold an impromptu CoDA group meeting right there.

DRUGS OF ADDICTION

There is a cornucopia of misinformation about drugs out there. Some drug users chose to simply remain ignorant of it all and bury their heads in the sand and their brains in the drugs. They deflect the adverse consequences of drug use with such cavalier statements as:

> *"Yeah, I know it's bad but something's gotta kill you, right?"* [At 19 years old?]

> *"I may as well die happy."* [Right next to this dumpster]

> *"I'm going to quit soon."* [As soon as my probation officer does my drug screen]

All that ridiculopathy aside, there is another confounding factor in getting the message to addicts. That confounder is the ever-present street pharmacologist whose wealth of pseudo-information and partial-truths is staggering. Akin to the street pharmacologist/jackass is the bathtub chemist who makes "pure" meth or "pure" LSD or "pure" XTC or "pure" whatever. Generally it's "pure" crap, but you will never get the addict to admit that. Then again it is hard to talk while you are having a seizure.

Most people in the "real world" are not that interested in the drug de jour or for that matter any other addictive drugs. They have no need to spend hours upon hours digging through mazes of neuro-psycho-pharmacological research unless they have a passion for it. I happen to have that passion, and I want to share some pragmatic information with you. Plus, I figure if you picked this book up, and if you've gotten this far into it, you will probably find this stuff pretty interesting.

There is one important fact to keep in mind as we talk about the various mood-altering/mood-addicting drugs. ALL of these drugs ultimately share a common pathway of addiction. This pathway connects the reward centers of the brain. It's called the mesocortico/mesolimbic and nigrostriatal systems, but we're going to stick with calling it the reward system.

If you have the brain disease of addiction, some of the long-lasting drug induced alterations that occur within your reward system actually involve changing the way your brain reads your own DNA. DNA is who you are. Addiction changes us.

That is why family members frequently tell me, *"We just want the old Donna back. She is a wonderful person, but the drugs have changed her."* Indeed they have.

Notice that I said addiction changes the way your body reads your DNA: it does not change your DNA. The science of epigenetics is a relatively new frontier of alcohol research. It is the study of changes in gene function that occur without changing the body's genetic code. Toxic substances and drugs can alter the way your body reads DNA which means your reward centers and brain chemicals (neurotransmitters) can be pathologically altered. You develop sick circuits. There is another scary part to this process. These changes can be transmitted from one generation to the next. Very scary!

The good news is that you can break away from the pathological thinking process of addiction. You can override the diseased circuits and develop healthy circuits that afford you a chance for a fulfilling life. It takes work and you have got to want it. It usually comes down to this rather stark question, "Are you sick and tired of being sick and tired?"

Only you really know the answer to that.

The next sections of this book deal with scientific facts about alcohol and other drugs.

DRUGS OF ADDICTION
Alcohol

Alcohol is still number one. Alcohol kills 6.5 times the number of people under 21 years old than all other addictive drugs combined.

Alcohol and Adolescents - What happens when you put a neurotoxic substance into a developing brain? First off, you get the immediate effect of brain dysfunction which is hopefully temporary. However, you may also get pathological brain development especially if the intake of the toxic drug continues.

The distinction between brain development and brain change is a pertinent one. A normally developed adult brain can be changed by addictive chemicals, but it will try to return to normal once the chemicals are gone (metabolized). If drug use starts at an early age, the user does not get a normally developed brain. Brain development that uses the artificial emotions created by drugs as its template becomes a mal-developed brain. If you start drugging and/or drinking at age thirteen, fourteen, or fifteen years old, you don't get a normal brain! You have no normal to go back to. You have to stop using the drugs in order for your brain to develop some semblance of normalcy.

As an aside, the brain is not a fully developed adult brain until after age twenty-five or perhaps on out to thirty years old. Choose wisely.

Alcohol is one of the toxic drugs that can cause brain mal-development. The developing brain of an adolescent does not handle alcohol the same way as a developed brain does. Adolescents tend to be able to drink more ethanol prior to sedation, and they have less of a "hangover" effect than adults. This is not a good thing as it promotes greater intake and greater toxic damage. The typical adolescent alcohol abuser is a binge drinker. A binge can adversely impact the brain for weeks and decrease learning ability during that time.

Alcohol alters the trajectory of brain development. Indeed, the adolescent binger may end up with the frontal parts of his or her brain smaller than that of the non-drinkers. That frontal part, called the prefrontal cortex, is what we use to make appropriate decisions and fit into family and society. It is what makes us mature and responsible.

It is not much of a leap to understand that if a person starts drinking at an early age and damages his prefrontal brain lobes and keeps drinking, he is going to have something akin to an adolescent brain when he is thirty years old. Can you imagine being married to such a guy? We used to call it "Peter Pan Syndrome" because this is a guy who never wants to grow up. He may be fun to be around and witty and happy go lucky. His wife may even refer to him as her "other child." Cute, huh? However, he will also be impaired when it comes to performing goal-directed behavior, like holding down a job. By the way, good luck on getting child support from Peter.

The same thing can happen with female adolescent drinkers only they get labeled as "Cinderellas" or "Princesses." Take it from there.

Alcoholically damaged adolescent brains, like these, cannot be rehabilitated because they were never normal. They must be habilitated.

The neurotoxic drug, alcohol, disrupts all sorts of brain chemicals (neurotransmitters), and that results in abnormal thinking. In most cases, I can't just look at you and know you have a damaged brain, but if I chat with you and talk to some family members, I can usually detect said damage.

What might I look for?

For discussion purposes, let's say you are a fifty-six-year-old "functional alcoholic." By functional, I mean you are married and you hold down a job. Your ritual is to come home and quietly get "blotto" every night. The family has learned to sort of work their lives out around you. You have no real concept of all the things you are missing out on. For instance, you don't even realize that your daughter won't let the grandkids call you after five o'clock. You surely don't realize that as they grow, your grandchildren will be told alcoholism runs in the family – "like Papa."

Your damaged brain interferes with your social interaction even when you are dry. This will be especially apparent with strangers, such as the fiancé your son brought home for the family to meet.

Social interaction requires you to understand what others are thinking in order for you to determine their mental state so that you can predict how they will react to you. In short, you need to be able to understand where other people are coming from. You also need to be able to interpret facial expressions and project your own appropriate facial expressions to others. You need to be able to empathize with others' emotions and share yours appropriately.

Alcohol use impairs the parts of your brain that direct appropriate social interaction. In other words, the part of your brain that keeps you from saying stupid things is broken. Your "social brakes" are not working so you say non-endearing things.

Son: *"Mom, Dad, this is Caroline, my girlfriend."*

Dad (alcoholic): *"Charlotte you say. No, wait a minute that was the other girlfriend. Well, I hope the hell he does not get you pregnant because he damn sure cannot afford a kid."*

Other brain areas that are susceptible to ethanol brain damage can result in alcohol dementia. It always saddens me to treat a fifty-something year old alcoholic with dementia.

Karen who is thirty years old, sat in my office and tearfully said this of her wine-drinking mother who recently left the stove on and was passed out on the couch when the firemen arrived. *"It is like she just does not seem to get it anymore. We do not dare leave the grandchildren with her and it is getting to where we do not even want them to see her, in that state of hers. She has chosen the wine over her family and her health. My husband talked to a lawyer friend of his. We are thinking about having her declared incompetent and putting her away somewhere safe. "*

Demented alcoholics can sit on the porch and drink beer all day with their other alcoholic buddies, and at the end of the day, they have little idea as to what was said. They are rude and inconsiderate of family members. They see everyone else as over-reacting. They act impulsively and say hurtful things. They fall down and hurt themselves. They get all sorts of medical problems from drinking, but they keep on drinking. They resist efforts of family members to make them stop drinking. They make empty promises and they lie about keeping them. They are often sneaky about drinking and may resort to hiding booze.

Stephen is a fifty-five-year-old male who presented to my office with the following history as related to me by his wife. "He and his so-called friends get *drunk every day, and four months ago he fell and broke his hip. He ended up in ICU because he had Dts, and the doctors told me they did not know if he would live or die. He does not remember any of that. I was by his side night and day praying that he would live and get better and not drink any more. He went to physical rehab, and then as soon as he got home he started drinking again. I find alcohol everywhere, even in the back of the commode. He has gotten to where he says mean things to me all the time. We have been married thirty-one years, but I have had it. It is killing me. I cannot lift him up off the floor anymore. I am moving to Mississippi to live with my daughter until he gets sober for good or I am gone for good."*

Stephen's version which he relates to me when we are alone is somewhat different. "Yes, I fell but I was trying to change a light, and the damn folding chair broke. I do not remember much of the hospital, but I got a new hip and I can get around. Hell, let her go. She runs my friends off anyway, and besides that I can take care of myself. I can stop any time I want."

Stephen elected not to seek treatment. His wife moved away and has no plans of ever coming back. She has started a new life and is enjoying her grandchildren. Stephen was found unconscious in his house. The electricity had been off for weeks. The water was also turned off, and he was living in filth. He had a severe infection to both lower legs along with severe liver cirrhosis. A CT scan of his brain showed generalized shrinking most prominent in the prefrontal lobes. His brain disease progressed to the point of satisfying the definition for being "gravely disabled." He now resides in a low-end nursing home.

Alcohol Withdrawal Syndrome - If Stephen had made the right decision, which was to enter treatment, he might have avoided such a horrible fate. Given his level of use (drinking all day) and his medical problems (high blood pressure, pancreatitis, liver disease, nerve damage to his legs, generalized muscle deconditioning), he would have required medical detoxification. He was at high risk for alcohol withdrawal complications such as a heart attack, a fatal heart rhythm, stroke, or a hemorrhage from his gastrointestinal tract, seizures, or a bunch more things nobody wants.

The brain adapts to having a sedating drug such as alcohol on board by increasing its neuro-electrical activity. The brain is actually trying to compensate for the sedating effects of alcohol because the brain always seeks internal balance (homeostasis). Alcohol disrupts this balance.

If I stay intoxicated, my brain will compensate by gearing up. If I stop drinking abruptly, my brain is still geared up and is in a hyperactive state, but since there is no longer any alcohol to offset the hyperactive state, the electrical and chemical activity in my brain goes wild.

This uncontrolled hyperactive brain state is called the Alcohol Withdrawal Syndrome, and it can kill you. The hyperactivity shows up as severe anxiety, shakiness, seizures, hallucinations, and more brain damage. The goal of a good medical detox is to "stay ahead of the detox curve" which means treat the symptoms before or as soon as they occur. Once you get behind, it is much harder to catch up because the damage has accelerated.

The main excitatory chemical causing this detrimental brain hyperactivity is glutamate. Too much glutamate causes a lot of problems, not the least of which is more brain damage. We want to keep it as normalized as possible. To do this, we give the patient a sedative and we adjust the dose to stabilize the brain. Once the brain is stabilized, we gradually withdraw the sedative in a controlled and monitored manner.

Of course, glutamate is not the only brain chemical that is out of whack. The natural sedative (GABA) in the brain is depleted by drinking. This depletion promotes severe anxiety and seizures when the alcoholic stops drinking alcohol. Dopamine, norepinephrine, serotonin and others are also out of balance.

Medical detox is usually not simple or straightforward with chronic alcoholics, at least not my alcoholics. Frequently, there are other medical problems that must be monitored and stabilized. Alcoholics are often on "fall precautions" for a variety of reasons. They are often malnourished (even though they might not look it), and one of the most important things to give them is thiamine also called Vitamin B1. Thiamine is somewhat protective of brain and nerve damage that can accompany alcohol withdrawal. I might not be able to repair the damage that is already done, but I can hopefully stop or slow down ongoing damage by prompt and adequate treatment.

During acute alcohol withdrawal, the main medications I rely upon are benzodiazepines. I prescribe the short-acting benzodiazepine oxazepam (Serax) for some patients, and I prescribe the long acting benzodiazepine chlordiazepoxide (Librium) for other patients. Both have advantages and disadvantages. It is important to match the right type of medication to the needs and condition of the patient.

Untreated Alcohol Withdrawal Syndrome - When a chronic drinker abruptly stops all intake of alcohol, a clinically predictable chain of events follows. There are even therapeutic tools called Alcohol Withdrawal Scales or AWS's that map out the signs and symptoms of alcohol withdrawal and rate their level of severity. Based upon the AWS score, the tool may be matched with guidelines for medication doses. These scales should strictly be used as guidelines. I do not rely upon them because I prefer individualized treatment rather than cookie cutter therapy.

Signs and Symptoms of Acute Alcohol Withdrawal - Upon abrupt cessation of alcohol intake in a physiologically dependent person, a relatively predictable chain of events occurs. Generally, the person starts to feel anxious a few hours after the last drink. The person may also start to have hand tremors, sweats, nausea, and insomnia. Pulse and blood pressure go up. Now is the time to begin medication for alcohol withdrawal. It is clinically noteworthy that an alcoholic may have a blood alcohol level above "legal intoxication" and still be in overt withdrawal and in need of medication.

Without adequate treatment, some patients report hallucinations within a day of stopping the alcohol. They are aware that these auditory, visual, or skin perceptions are not real. It's call alcoholic hallucinosis. (This is not "DTs.")

> *When I was in detox in 1978, one of my roommates was a "real" alcoholic. He looked the part too. He had that ruddy facial complexion and scars on his face from various encounters of the cement kind. He was one of those big construction worker types who liked to fight when he got drunk. He was a nice enough guy sober, though. He was in the bed next to mine, and he would lie there and describe his visual hallucinations. I remember him vividly describing a tiger crouched on top of the wardrobe and telling me not to worry because it was friendly. Well, you can imagine that he scared the hell out of me and I am not talking about the tiger; I never saw him; I am talking about my roommate.*

If the detoxing alcoholic is going to have seizures, they usually start within twenty-four to forty-eight hours. However, I have seen it happen as late as five days after stopping. Seizures are dangerous for several reasons, including fall injuries, but they are usually self-limiting. This means they stop on their own. Sadly, that is not always the case and there is a condition called status epilepticus in which you constantly seizure until your body exhausts out, and you die a rather ignoble death.

DTs (Delirium Tremens) can start after a day or two and this is a life-threatening situation. The person is severely disoriented. Blood pressure may skyrocket, and there is the risk of stroke. The heart may beat rapidly and abnormally and there is the risk of a fatal cardiac event. The person can become dehydrated, and this makes matters even more critical. When things get this far out of control, the patient needs to be admitted to a medical hospital.

DTs are relatively rare in a treatment center for several reasons. For one thing, we know our patients are alcoholics. For another, we know how to watch out for early development of withdrawal, and we can generally control it and prevent DTs. This may not be the case in a general hospital. The patient may not let anyone know about his drinking when he goes to the hospital for a broken leg. He goes off to surgery and has the leg repaired, and then 48 hours later he is strapped to a bed having DTs because no one knew to treat him for alcohol withdrawal until then.

The best treatment for an alcohol withdrawal syndrome is prevention. I do not endorse waiting until the person is in full-blown alcohol withdrawal to start benzodiazepines. That used to be called "earning your detox meds." I think that is poor practice if not malpractice. Based upon the nursing and addictionology assessments, I titrate the patient to a safe medication level, keep him there a day or two, then I decrease the medication over five-to-seven days as clinically tolerated.

There are clinical clues that can help predict the severity of the withdrawal process. For example, it is very important to inquire about the patient's past medical history as it relates to alcohol withdrawal. Repeated bouts of drinking and detoxing cause the brain to become super-sensitive to alcohol withdrawal. This is called the 'kindling effect." This super-sensitivity phenomenon results in progressive worsening of the severely of the alcohol withdrawal syndromes.

> *"I used to be able to detox off alcohol on my own. I would go to the camp with a couple of fifths and drink less and less over a few days until I ran out. Then I would get the sweats and the shakes, but I could get though it after a few days. The last time I tried that, I ended up having a seizure, and my heart started beating real funny. I ended up in a little hospital down on the bayou. They took good care of me, though. A young doctor there told me I was lucky I did not die at the camp. Of course, that did not stop me and I got back on the sauce. So, I decided to come to detox last night because I was scared to try to do it by myself again. But I have got to stop. This is killing me. My last drink was at the gate here."* Oscar is a 46-year-old car salesman who drove himself to treatment in a company car. His drug of choice is alcohol. He has a history of multiple detoxifications. His breathalyzer is twice the legal limit for impairment, but he exhibits no obvious signs of intoxication.

The initial blood tests that I get on an alcoholic patient can be very important indicators of the severity of his ethanol dependency. For instance if his red blood cells are enlarged, I know he is a chronic heavy drinker, no matter what he might think or tell me. It also signals a B vitamin deficiency that, if left untreated, can result in brain and nerve damage.

I'm going to expand on one particularly important B vitamin in alcoholism. That vitamin is **thiamine** or **B1.** If you are going to treat alcoholics, it is very important that you understand the relationship between thiamine and alcohol dependency. A severe deficiency of vitamin B1 can occur rapidly in alcoholics. This is especially true of alcoholics who have undergone weight-loss surgery and are drinking. Whatever the cause, low vitamin B1 can result in a condition called Wernicke's Encephalopathy. This is a true medical emergency with a twenty percent fatality rate if you don't treat it right away. Clinicians are trained to look for the triad of (1) abnormal or decreased eye movement (2) staggering gait and muscle incoordination (3) confusion and difficulty thinking. Counselors are generally not trained to look for Wernicke's which is unfortunate since up to eighty percent of the cases are not diagnosed until late in the process, and time lost equals brain lost. An astute therapist with a high index of suspicion could conceivably recognize the problem and refer the patient to medical personnel for immediate treatment.

Inappropriate medical care can actually push an alcoholic into Wernicke's. This can be the result of abruptly increasing the patient's carbohydrate load without giving vitamin B1 to compensate for that load. How does this happen? If we give an alcoholic with a low vitamin B1 level a high carbohydrate load, the increase in sugar causes a sudden decrease of vitamin B1. An IV infusion of glucose (dextrose) is a high carb load. So, giving an alcoholic a plain IV bag of glucose can result in brain damage and/or death. That is why we always add minerals and vitamins including thiamine to the IV bags we give to active alcoholics. The vitamins make the solution yellow, so we call them banana bags.

Early treatment of Wernicke's can stop the progression of the brain damage and promote some recovery. Untreated Wernicke's can progress to Korsakoff's Psychosis.

The hallmark of Korsakoff's Syndrome is severe memory problems. Memory loss is often extreme, and the person cannot form new memories. We used to see these patients wandering about the backwards of state psychiatric hospitals. My first encounter with a Korsakoff patient occurred on the third floor of Charity Hospital of New Orleans (CHNO). I was a junior at LSU Medical School at the time, and the dreaded third floor was the locked psychiatric ward. The patient was a man in his mid-fifties who was "assigned" to me on my psych rotation. I introduced myself to him, and I found him cordial, but he told me that he did not feel comfortable discussing business in the hallway. He went on to give me this great story of how he was a business executive, and this was his office building and then invited me into his office. He was oblivious to the fact that he was in a psych ward, dressed in state-issue pajamas, and pointing to the dayroom as his office. There is a name for making up stories like that to fill in the gaps. This is called confabulation. Poor guy, he never spent another day outside of an institution.

There are other lab tests that I routinely order in patients with an alcohol withdrawal syndrome. Platelets help clot our blood if we start bleeding. Low platelets in an alcoholic are of special significance since the person might bleed more easily than normal. For instance, in the case of very low platelets, a seizure and a fall could result in a brain hemorrhage. Low potassium levels are dangerous in that the heart needs normal potassium to beat properly. Low potassium can kill you. Low potassium is also a predictor that the alcoholic is going to have a hard detox. A high ammonia level means severe liver disease, and it also means I will use a short-acting benzodiazepine for this patient because he or she can't metabolize the long-acting benzodiazepine with an impaired liver. Plus, since a high ammonia level clouds the mind, the longer acting benzodiazepine will cloud the mind even more. Like I said, I do not like cookie cutter, "routine" detox orders. There are other factors to consider, but I think we all get the picture.

Acute detox usually lasts five to seven days if we get ahead of it. However, after the acute phase, it is not uncommon to have mental cloudiness, memory problems, concentration problems, anxiety, depression, sleep problems, and low frustration tolerance. This is all part of the post-acute alcohol withdrawal syndrome. The symptoms are worse in the first four to eight weeks but continue to get better over time. It may take over a year or two to get back to one's normal baseline. There are some mental exercises that can help. Of course, if one drinks, he or she goes right back to ground zero.

Blood Alcohol Levels- Since there seems to be a global misconception about blood alcohol levels, I want to spend a little time on the topic. Almost everyone knows 0.8 is the "legal level" of intoxication. At that level, if a person is driving a vehicle, he or she is officially impaired and is in criminal violation of the law.

Unfortunately, this legal administrative number tends to make people think that if their blood alcohol concentration (BAC) is less than 0.8, they are "all right." This is scientifically proven to be irrefutably not true. If you have any alcohol on board when you get behind the wheel, you are impaired. That is the simple truth of the matter.
The message we send out with this legal definition is that we, as a society, say it is okay to drive with an alcohol concentration of 0.079! This is what we are telling society,

and more importantly this is the message we give to our children. We as a nation, via our government, know this is not true. I say this without reservation because according to Federal Law, administered by the Department of Transportation (DOT), if a commercial truck driver has an alcohol concentration of 0.02 or more, that driver is taken off the road. The number 0.02 equates to one beer or one glass of wine. Why does DOT do this? It is a scientific fact that at 0.02 BAC or above there is measurable impairment of driving-related skills.

For truck drivers, who are experienced, trained, and hold a commercial license, the USA says they are impaired at a 0.02 BAC, but the rest of the drivers in America are okay until they reach almost four times that level! This simply makes no sense at all to me as a citizen or a clinician.

There is more worth noting about that DOT law. If a driver has an alcohol concentration of 0.04 or more, he or she must go for an evaluation by a substance-abuse professional or SAP. Why does DOT do this? At a BAC of 0.04, all measures of driving skills are significantly impaired. If that driver wants to maintain a commercial license, he or she must follow whatever that SAP says to do. After completing the SAP's recommendations for education and/or treatment, that driver must have a least twelve months follow up which will include at least six random drug and alcohol tests by a DOT approved lab.

This DOT example is a blatant indicator that the current 0.08 BAC level is not based upon sound scientific information or research. Indeed it is quite the opposite as it flies in the face of scientific data. This is a serious situation. In fact, it is so serious that the National Transportation Safety Board, or NTSB, is pushing to drop the level of legal intoxication to 0.05 BAC. At 0.05, the risk on having an accident increases by forty percent, even if the level goes to 0.05, we are still condoning driving while impaired!

We would all be a lot safer with the legal limit at 0.05 but not as safe as if we followed the DOT level of 0.20 BAC as the cutoff.

The glaring fact here is that the safest call would be zero tolerance.

The NTSB states that by lowering the BAC to 0.05, we could prevent almost 1000 deaths, caused by intoxicated drivers, per year. We could prevent intoxicated drivers from killing three people a day! That number of lives saved is based in part upon what has happened in other countries, like Australia, which dropped the legal BAC to 0.05.

Do not expect any of this to happen soon. NTSB is getting plenty of pushback from the alcohol and hospitality industry. It took years and plenty of death and trauma to get all the states to agree to drop the legal intoxication level from 0.10 to 0.8!

Clinical vs. Forensic Blood Alcohol Level Measurements-
Since patients have asked me about this, I want to clarify some things about the alcohol breath test we do if you come to detox. This is not a legal or forensic test. It can never be used as a forensic result because neither the testing instrument nor the procedure meets forensic standards. This is not a legal test. As a matter of fact, due to strict confidentiality laws, no one can even know you are at detox unless you want them to know, and no one can get your records unless you specifically release them.

The breath test we do is a clinical tool to let us know if you have tolerance to alcohol. In short we need to know your alcohol concentration (BAC) and how it affects you. If your BAC is 0.13, and you have a no signs or symptoms of intoxication, we immediately know that you have a high tolerance and that we will probably need to give you medications to help you detox safely. If you BAC is 0.37 and you seem drunk, we need to closely monitor you for acute problems such as vomiting and sucking it into your lung. Then we will check your BAC periodically as you detox and use that as a guide for the medications you may require. Clinical BAC tests are about keeping patients safe.

Medications for Alcohol Dependency

Since addiction is a physical brain disease caused by mood-altering chemicals, it is logical that other chemicals in the form of medications could be developed to treat this disease. Such research is ongoing, and there have been medical advances in the addiction field. As such, we do have some medications that can assist in the recovery process.

Substance use disorders or addictions are due to malfunctions and mal-development of brain chemicals and brain circuits. This is the biological basis of addiction. Once the addiction is biologically established, social, psychological, and spiritual dysfunctions ensue.

There are medications that can help re-establish or establish healthy, functional brain circuits as well as healthy brain chemical balances. These medications help the brain normalize. They do not fix the addicted brain. They do not fix the social, psychological or spiritual malfunctions. These medications as a whole decrease craving and decrease the pleasurable effects of addictive drugs and/or behaviors. The operative word is "decrease"!

In order to rehabilitate or habilitate an addicted brain, the recovering addict must practice healthy behaviors to establish and strengthen healthy brain circuits. The dysfunctionally addicted brain circuits do not go away, but the development and reinforcement of healthy brain circuits will weaken the addicted circuits and can in essence silence them.

Since the addicted circuits may never go away, it is as though the addict has an allergy to addictive drugs and can reactivate the unhealthy, addicted circuits by using addictive drugs. This is why addiction is referred to as a chronic disease prone to relapse. If the recovering addict does not continue to reinforce healthy brain circuits, the unhealthy ones can take over again.

<u>Medications help. They do not cure.</u>

DISCLAIMER

I am about to talk about some of the medications used to stabilize the addicted brain and to help decrease craving and to treat co-existing disorders. Sadly, in our current state of societal affairs I must insert the following since I have found that on occasion my grandfather was right when he told me that no good deed goes unpunished.

Disclaimer: The opinions I express about these medications are just that – my opinions. This is not medical advice. Any decision to take any medication must be made by the patient and his or her physician or other legal prescriber. I do not have any stock or financial interest in any drug company, and I am not promoting any medication. I am presenting this information to assist the addict in knowing what medications are available. This is an overview or summary, and it is intended to give the addict an overview of what medication is available to help in recovery. This is not individual medical advice. Some of these medications are used "off label," and I am not suggesting that anyone else do that.

If you are considering getting a prescription for any of these medications, get with your healthcare professional. The medications may not be suitable or appropriate for you and/or your situation. Always, as in ALWAYS, be informed about what you are taking. This goes for any medication. Read the package insert and patient information. Ask your pharmacist for information. It is not possible to present an all-inclusive list of what side effects might happen in this relatively short overview.

Disulfiram for Alcohol Dependency

Disulfiram's trade name is Antabuse. It is available as a generic medication. While it was initially envisioned for the treatment of alcohol abuse only, it seems to have some promise for use in cocaine addiction and compulsive gambling.

Disulfiram has been around a long time. Indeed, its adverse interaction with alcohol was discovered by chance. Disulfiram was used in the vulcanization process for rubber long before it was recognized as a medication that could help treat alcoholism. In 1937, a plant physician wrote a medical article about how workers who were exposed to disulfiram at the rubber plant were getting sick when they drank alcohol. His article evidently disappeared into the black hole of academentia as nothing more became of it. (What a missed opportunity that was.)

Then, around 1945 two scientists were testing the drug as a treatment for intestinal worms. It seemed to work well on rabbits afflicted with intestinal parasites. (That would be non-drinking rabbits). As the story goes, these two scientists took the medication themselves (as was the custom in those days) to see if there were any adverse effects. Things seemed okay until they separately drank alcohol. One had "a beer" and had a light reaction. The other evidently was planning to do what we would call "partying" today but got very sick instead. (Oops!) They later compared experiences, and being the scientists they were figured it best not to drink with that particular worm medicine on board.

A few years later (1948), a psychiatrist decided to use it as "aversion therapy." He would give the alcoholics Antabuse and have them drink alcohol. They would get porcelain hugging sick and that was the goal of treatment. Actually, that was the treatment. The idea was that after a while the alcoholic would associate alcohol with being sick and have an aversion to it. Little did he know how powerful alcohol is to an alcoholic.

Can you imagine how desperate an alcoholic would be to submit to a course of torture in hopes of getting "a cure"? (Some of us can.) To this doctor's credit, he decided that aversion therapy was not enough by itself and realized psychological therapy was also needed. Subsequently, Antabuse became an adjunct medication and was approved for the treatment of alcoholism.

Just for reference, Alcoholics Anonymous had been around for roughly fifteen years when all this was taking place.

How Antabuse Works:
When a person drinks "beverage alcohol" which is ethanol, the ethanol is broken down or "metabolized" in the following manner:

1. Ethanol is metabolized into acetaldehyde by an enzyme called alcohol dehydrogenase.
2. The acetaldehyde is then metabolized into acetic acid (which is harmless) by an enzyme called acetaldehyde dehydrogenase.
3. Disulfiram (Antabuse) blocks this part of the metabolism by blocking the acetaldehyde dehydrogenase enzyme.
4. There is a buildup of acetaldehyde to toxic levels.
5. This makes the drinker "sick as a dog."

How sick as a dog? Well, you feel hot, your skin flushes, you have a throbbing headache, your heart rate jumps up, you get nausea and vomiting, you may get very dizzy and even faint when you try to stand up, you may get confused, and you may even have your circulatory system collapse. It's sort of like a super hangover with no initial high, except this hangover can be very dangerous especially if you have any heart or circulation problems.

If you take Antabuse and ingest ethanol, you are going to get pretty sick pretty quickly. I have treated Antabuse-alcohol reactions in the emergency room, and it is not a pretty sight. Here is a composite case history:

> *Herman is a 44-year-old male who presents to the emergency room with a chief complaint of: "I think I'm having a heart attack." Upon initial examination it is noted that his face is very flushed. He is very anxious and sweating profusely. He complains that he cannot catch his breath. His pulse rate is 120 beats per minute. He vomits into the trash can during the initial assessment. His history is positive for alcoholism. He tells me he had been on Antabuse but stopped it two days ago so he could drink. He goes on to say, "I only took one damn drink and I started getting sick within ten minutes. How stupid can I get?" Well, the obvious answer is "Pretty stupid!" I refrain from expressing that particular opinion. After all, it is a cunning and powerful brain disease. He is given oxygen, IV fluids, and thiamine. His nausea is treated with Zofran. We could also give massive doses of Vitamin C but that is not indicated here. Luckily, he did not have any permanent consequences from his disulfiram-ethanol-reaction (DER). In extreme cases, shock, coma, and/or death can occur. As for the social consequences of his behavior, his wife, an Al-Anon member, provided most of those.*

Dosage: Today, a common course of therapy would be to give 500 mg per day for a week or so then drop the dose to 250 mg per day. It is odorless and practically tasteless. It can be crushed and dissolved in water. The alcoholic must be totally dry for at least twelve hours before taking Antabuse. I prefer at least three days of abstinence prior to initiation of this medication.

How long do I take it? Disulfiram can be taken for months to years with appropriate medical follow up. It is not a cure but can help the alcoholic get into a recovery process.

Disulfiram can also help an alcoholic get through high risk situations.

> *Bob is an alcoholic with a couple of month's sobriety. His father died, and Bob must fly from Louisiana to some remote place in Oregon for the funeral. Bob is already thinking about the booze on the plane and the booze at the airport terminal bar and the booze that will flow at the wake. He is nervous about all these triggers to drink, and he is worried about getting thirsty. He meets with his addictionologist, and they decide that Antabuse will offer him some security from relapse. He plans to take it for one week then stop taking it when he gets back home and back into his support system. Of course, he plans to call his sponsor daily, when he can, while on the trip.*

Does it work? Research shows that disulfiram does work in alcoholics who are motivated and willing to get into a recovery process. It also affords some comfort to the co-dependent as it decreases the likelihood of getting the dreaded knock on the door at 3:00 a.m. If you have this disease and have someone who cares about you, you should know exactly what I mean when I refer to "the knock on the door." If you are the co-dependent, you definitely know what I mean.

Some of the side effects may include the following:
- Disulfiram may interact with other medications you

are taking. A complete medical evaluation is needed prior to prescribing this medication.

- Decreased energy or "tiredness" and even drowsiness may occur. These should decrease within a short period of time. You might want to take the disulfiram at night if it causes these side effects.
- A garlicky or metallic taste in the mouth occurs in some people. This usually goes away in about two weeks.
- Headaches may occur initially but should go away within short time.
- Impotency (uncommon) may occur in men. Needless to say, whenever I bring this up, I have some males who do not want to take disulfiram for this very reason. And, I have some wives who want them to take disulfiram for this very reason. After all, who wants to have sex with a drunk, except maybe another drunk? While this adverse effect is uncommon it is a serious effect and the physician needs to be notified immediately as it may indicate adverse neurological effects.
- Other serious side effects that can occur include but are not limited to neurological changes, liver problems, muscle weakness, gastrointestinal problems, and/or allergic reactions.
- LET YOUR PHYSICIAN/PRESCRIBER KNOW OF ANY SIDE EFFECTS IMMEDIATELY.

Disulfiram toxicity is uncommon today. When the drug was first approved, some patients were given 3000 mg per day! Disulfiram toxicity can be fatal due to organ system failure.

Pros & Cons & Comments: Antabuse does not appear to impact craving. Its use is considered aversion therapy. Think of Antabuse therapy as an *"if you use, you lose"* sort of thing, except in this case you get so sick that everyone knows you lose. Of course, hidden alcohol such as that in a rum cake could trigger the reaction. Then again, any alcoholic in recovery should know to avoid "hidden alcohol." Your prescriber and/or pharmacist should give you a "how to list" for taking disulfiram. If not, ask for one. (As an aside, I did include a note about alcohol and cooking in the glossary.)

This medication generally needs to be taken daily. In some cases, it is beneficial to have a family member witness the ingestion of the medication. This is something that needs to be worked out in a therapist's office as this can breed resentment and the like. Antabuse is not a cure, but it can buy the alcoholic some dry time. Dry time is defined as taking in no alcohol. By the way, an alcoholic is not dry if he or she is taking an alcohol substitute such as Xanax, Ativan, Valium, or Klonopin. All these benzodiazepines equate to alcohol in pill form for the alcoholic. The effects of Antabuse can last for days and even for up to two weeks following discontinuation of the medication. It is not addictive.

A Cautionary Tale to Co-dependents: I had one of my male patients tell me that his wife slipped Antabuse into his food one evening. She did this because she thought he was lying about not drinking. She was right. After he left the hospital, he was thinking about having her arrested for attempted murder. The moral of the story is simple: do not secretly give Antabuse to an alcoholic. Planting Antabuse in beverages or food is a practice to be absolutely condemned. Nobody wins if the alcoholic ends up in a hospital or morgue, and the co-dependent ends up in jail and the kids in a foster home. Enough said.

Disulfiram use in cocaine dependency and compulsive gambling is presented under separate headings.

Acamposate for Alcohol Dependency

Acamposate's trade name is Campral. It is used to decrease craving and improve abstinence from alcohol. Alcoholism, alcohol withdrawal, and especially important, alcohol craving are associated with an imbalance of a brain chemical named "glutamate." We talked a little about this earlier. Glutamate can cause over-excitability of nerve cells. This is not a good thing as this over-excitement may cause nerve-cell damage, severe anxiety, and panic attacks. The action of acamposate is to decrease the over activity of glutamate and thereby decrease the over-excitability that is causing the damage, anxiety, and/or panic. Please note, acamposate is not a treatment for the alcohol withdrawal syndrome. Acamposate also has some impact on another brain chemical called GABA which is essentially the body's own internal benzodiazepine. GABA helps control anxiety. Therefore Acamposate's action on GABA plays a role in controlling anxiety and hyper-excitability.

There is some indication that acamposate is more effective in more severe alcoholics, but any alcoholic has the potential to benefit from acamposate. Simply put, it works for some people but not for others. There appears to be no real way to know which alcoholic will benefit from acamposate. It has few side effects, so a trial of the medication might be warranted in any alcoholic who has cravings and/or relapses.

Dosage: Take two 333 mg tablets three times a day. Acamposate can be taken with meals to help you remember to take it.

It can be started during or after detoxification. It can even be taken while the person is intoxicated. There is no adverse reaction when this is done.

Acamposate should generally be taken for twelve months. However, if there is no response such as decreased craving and/or decreased alcohol drinking after four to six weeks, there is no reason to continue acamposate. Interestingly, the positive effects of acamposate may persist for three to twelve months after the person stops taking a course of treatment.

Side Effects: The main side effects are gastrointestinal such as intestinal gas (which may have a negative social impact), diarrhea, "upset stomach", and/or decreased appetite. It could cause mental confusion, dizziness, and/or drowsiness. People with kidney disease should not take it. As with any drug, any body system can be adversely affected. Hence, there is need for medical monitoring.

Suicide: There is some indication that acamposate may increase the risk of suicide. I do not know why this is. I do know that most alcoholics are depressed by the situations they are in. Alcohol in and of itself has depressive effects. Some alcoholics have depression apart from the alcohol or the situation. I also know that "taking away alcohol" can cause somewhat of a grief response to losing the alcohol. There is also the possibility that the drinker was using the alcohol to "treat" his or her depression. Then there is the depression that comes with relapse. I do not have the answer. The bottom line is that increased suicide risk is associated with use of acamposate. This is infrequent, but if you get depressed and/or any family members or "concerned others" see you getting depressed, let your physician know about it.

In one study about acamposate, of 2272 alcoholics taking acamposate, three people committed suicide. In the comparison group of 1962 alcoholics not taking acamposate (but taking placebos or sugar pills), two people committed suicide.

Pros & Cons & Comments: Acamposate is not a stand-alone treatment for alcoholism. It is most beneficial when used with concurrent involvement in a recovery program. Even if you start drinking, you should continue to take acamposate. Taking acamposate while drinking seems to decrease the severity and the length of the relapse. There is less relapse in alcoholics taking acamposate, and there appears to be less craving. It only works in alcoholism. It does not impact taking other addictive drugs. There are minimal drug interactions with acamposate and that is a plus. Naltrexone may increase the concentration of acamposate in the blood. Some folks have a hard time remembering to take medication three times a day. All in all, acamposate may be worth a try in motivated alcoholics. Researchers have shown that it can double the abstinence rate among alcoholics one to two years after treatment. I have talked with some alcoholics who told me it did nothing, and others who told me it "knocked the edge off craving." The only real way to know if it will work for you is to try it. It is not addictive.

Naltrexone for Alcohol Dependency

Naltrexone comes in a form you can take by mouth (trade names ReVia & Depade) and in an injectable form (trade name Vivitrol). It is an opiate antagonist. This simply means it blocks the effect of opiate receptors in your brain. In other words, if you inject, inhale, or swallow an opiate, the opiate has no effect.

Interestingly, naltrexone is also beneficial in addicts whose drug of choice is alcohol. Alcohol drinking causes the natural opiates in your brain to be released in access. That is one of the reasons alcohol makes an alcoholic feel good. The point here is that if naltrexone blocks some of the good feelings an alcoholic might get from drinking alcohol, the alcoholic might not drink or at least not drink as much. The reasoning is that if alcohol is not producing the desired euphoria, why continue to drink?

The naltrexone effect may decrease the probability of a "lapse" turning into a "relapse." For our purposes the definition of a lapse, or slip, is a single drink or single drinking episode of very short duration. As such, a three-week binge is not a lapse.

Naltrexone may be helpful in alcoholism but it is not a cure-all. I wish recovery was that simple. It is not. Other brain chemicals, not affected by naltrexone, are at work in the alcoholic brain. These neurotransmitters promote compulsive alcohol drinking.

Naltrexone can be started prior to or during detoxification from alcohol. Most physicians start it after the alcoholic has dried out a little. There is some indication that naltrexone may decrease alcohol craving.

Dosage oral pill form: Generally, oral naltrexone is taken at a dose of 50 mg by mouth each day. There are other dosing regimens, but this is the most common one and probably the best way to go if using the oral form. If there is no positive effect within four to six weeks, you may as well stop it.

For attenuation of a drinking episode, naltrexone could be taken during a binge with the intent of decreasing the severity of the binge. Another way to take it would be only when craving alcohol.

There is no optimal length of time for taking naltrexone, but if it works, taking the medication for a month to a year seems reasonable. There may be a "carry over" beneficial effect for months after the drug is discontinued.

Dosage Intramuscular injection: The recommended dosage of injectable naltrexone (Vivitrol) is 380 mg injected into muscle tissue (that would be in the upper outer quadrant of your butt) every four weeks.

Does it work for alcoholics: Just as with everything else, naltrexone works for some alcoholics but not for others. It seems to work best in those alcoholics with a positive family history for alcoholism. Of course, if you don't have an alcoholic relative, you should not be excluded from giving it a try.

Naltrexone may dampen the alcohol high, but you can drink through that with a little dedication. Plus, there are always other drugs that naltrexone does not block, like benzodiazepines (Xanax, Klonopin), cocaine, amphetamines, marijuana, and "synthetic marijuana" and so on.

If your drug of choice is alcohol, naltrexone may help increase your chances of recovery.

There is also clinical support for using a combination of

gabapentin (Neurontin) and naltrexone in the treatment of alcoholism. This combination has been shown to decrease heavy drinking in alcoholics, and the combination of the two may be better than either of these drugs alone.

Adverse Side Effects: Liver damage is a concern with naltrexone albeit the injectable naltrexone is less prone to cause liver damage. There may be pain at the injection site with the naltrexone XR (Vivitrol). I insist that any addict I am going to inject with naltrexone XR has a complete understanding of the drug and its side effects. Of course, I do the same with oral naltrexone. Before injecting naltrexone, it may be a good idea to try an oral dose of naltrexone to make sure there are no adverse reactions. The injection is going to last for about four weeks, but the oral form can be stopped at any time and that is the end of it. There are other possible gastrointestinal side effects as well as effects on mood.

Naltrexone appears to be associated with an increase in testosterone levels.

Ondansetron (Zofran) Yes, this is an anti-nausea medication. However, it appears to decrease the dopamine surge induced by alcohol intake. Subsequently, there is less urge to drink and less incentive to continue drinking. It seems to work best on alcoholics who have an earlier onset of alcoholism. Prior to taking ondansetron, check for heart problems, do an ECG, and check liver functions as side effects can include cardiac and/or liver abnormalities, although these are uncommon.

Gabapentin (Neurontin) An anticonvulsant that may decrease craving, improve sleep, and decrease anxiety in alcoholics especially during the early day of sobriety. It may also decrease some obsessive compulsive type symptoms in alcoholics who suffer from such behaviors. In my patient population, I have observed mixed results. Gabapentin does have a therapeutic place in addiction treatment in some situations. As will be shown later in this book, I have noted some really good results with prescribing gabapentin to synthetic marijuana addicts. This medication may ultimately show greater benefit when combined with naltrexone.

Topiramate (Topamax) An anticonvulsant. Also used to treat migraine headaches. Topiramate may be beneficial in some alcoholics. It may decrease the desire to drink and/or decrease drinking episodes. Studies are still underway. The side effects can be significant, and ongoing monitoring, especially of kidney function, is important. Beside kidney problems, other side effects include eye problems, memory problems, and anorexia. Plus, topiramate can cause birth defects if taken during pregnancy. Interestingly, it may have a place in the treatment of obese patients with binge-eating disorders.

While my prescribing experience with this drug is limited, I have noted positive results from several patients. Topiramate may make detox a little less miserable, and patients have told me their craving levels have decreased while taking it. It is not a medication I would give someone a refillable prescription for because anyone taking it needs to have regular medical monitoring.

DRUGS OF ADDICTION
Opiates

Opium is actually a group of compounds that are produced by the opium poppy plant (Papaver somniferum) and have narcotic properties. The compounds are "alkaloids" which simply means they are naturally occurring or found in nature. Humans have been cultivating the opium plant in some form or another since the Neolithic Age (12,000 years ago), and there is some evidence that Neanderthal People used it 30,000 years ago. During our long history with the poppy plant, we have used it as a sacred religious vehicle, a medication, a poison, a means of suicide, a recreational drug, a food source, an oil source, and as a decorative plant. We have glorified it and demonized it. The Papaver somniferum plant grows to about two feet in height and has a pod on top of it the size of a hen's egg. This plant has played a major role in the pharmaceutical industry, as well as in other legal enterprises, illegal enterprises, wars, and world politics.

The term opiate refers to medication derived from the natural opium alkaloids. Morphine is an example. The term opioid refers to a synthetic medication that is by definition not derived from natural opium but has the same effects as opiates. Therefore, opioid is an all-inclusive term for narcotic pain medications.

The origin of the word narcotic means "to make numb." It certainly does that.

Opiates are used primarily as pain medications. Unfortunately, due to the ability of opiates to alter mood and cause euphoria, they are also highly addictive. Indeed, the exploitation of addicts by opium dealers has resulted in a host of medical and societal problems that even include warfare between nations.

The Anglo-Chinese Opium wars were fought between England and China in the 1800's. The wars were due to the fact that the Chinese government did not want England supplying opium to the Chinese citizenry. The Chinese realized opium smoking was a plague on their nation, and the British realized a lot of money could be made by supplying the drug. Subsequently, the Brits waged war and won access to Chinese ports and became International Drug dealers, and the Chinese suffered from widespread opium addiction and its consequences. The Brits also took a relatively small piece of Chinese real estate known as Hong Kong as part of the Opium War "treaty."

Opium, opiates, and opioids have continued to be "big business" with worldwide impact. The USA is the number one market for prescription opiates. Opiate use is pervasive in our nation. An attestation to the high prevalence of opioid use in the USA is that twenty percent of high school seniors in this county have taken opiates at least once in their lives.

Opiates act on the reward centers in your brain. They do this by locking on to special chemical receptors in your brain, especially one call the *"mu"* (pronounced mew like a kitty's meow) receptor. There are others opioid receptors, such as delta, kappa, and NOP that interact with opioids. Indeed, different opioids act differently on some of these receptors, but *mu* is the one that gives us the euphoria. *Mu* stimulation by opiates activates reward circuits. When these centers and circuits are activated, some people feel a tremendous euphoria. Some people report feeling as if all the stress and worries in their lives have been lifted and they can function. Some people feel a surge of energy, "like I can work forever." Some people feel tired or drugged, and they hate the feeling.

If you are one of the people who enjoys the feeling, you are at risk for addiction. With prolonged and compulsive use, addictive changes will occur within your brain. These changes can alter your thinking and your personality and therefore your behaviors. These changes can also make it very difficult for you to discontinue the use of opiates.

Many an addict has told me *"I hate who I have become now but I cannot seem to change."* Actually, you can change. The process is not easy, but it is certainly worth it.

There are plenty of different types of opiates available. Of course, heroin is ubiquitous but has no legal standing in the USA. Some of the opiate/opioid pain medications that can cause dependency with or without addiction are listed below. This list encompasses the opioids some of my addicted patients have reported to me as their drug(s) of choice. The common trade name is listed first and the generic name is in parenthesis.

> Demerol (meperidine)
> Dilaudid (hydromorphone)
> Duragesic (fentanyl)
> Lortab (hydrocodone)
> Dolophine (methadone
> MS Contin (morphine)
> Norco (hydrocodone)
> Opana (oxymorphone)
> Oxycontin (oxycodone)
> Percodan (oxycodone)
> Roxicodone (oxycodone)
> Suboxone, Subutex (buprenorphine)
> Zubsolv (buprenorphine)
> Ultram (Tramadol)
> Zohydro ER (a form of hydrocodone released 2013)

Ultram (tramadol) deserves special mention here because there seems to be some misunderstanding about it. It is an opioid. Tramadol was not a controlled drug initially, but it should have been. It was classified as controlled in 2014. Prior to being categorized as a controlled substance, it was listed as a "medication of concern." This means that tramadol prescriptions were being tracked by the Board of Pharmacy. It can cause physical dependency, and it can cause addiction. I have treated opiate addicts who use tramadol as their primary "drug of choice." Interestingly, high doses of Ultram can cause seizures.

Tramadol also has effects similar to some antidepressant medications. This means that if you mix regular antidepressant medications with tramadol, you can experience a severe, even life threatening reaction, called Serotonin Syndrome.

Withdrawal from tramadol is just like the detoxification from any other opiate listed above. However, some people who detox from tramadol get a psychosis characterized by hallucinations, paranoia, and mental confusion. There can also be increased suicidal ideation during withdrawal.

If you have the disease of addiction, you need to treat tramadol just as you would any other opiate. I have seen several opiate addicts relapse behind a tramadol prescription.

> *"You know, Doc. I figured it was only Ultram. I mean come on, Ultram; it is not like a real opiate. Anyway, I got some from my doctor for back pain. I admit they gave me a little boost, so I took the whole prescription in three days. Then I got to craving Roxies, and I took one and then I was back into it. I am snorting six Roxies a day, and my wife kicked me out. So here I am, back again all because of a stupid tramadol ride that sucked. I guess you were right; there is no free ride."* Timmy – readmitted for detoxification.

Dependency vs. Addiction: If a person takes opiates as prescribed on a regular basis for a week or two, he or she will develop a mild degree of tolerance and dependency. This does not make that person an addict. There may be some withdrawal that is relatively mild in nature when the medication is stopped. The non-addict has no problem complying with the medication directions or stopping the medication. Often times the non-addict has pills left over which he or she flushes down the drain. In addiction, there is dependency, but there is also chronic, compulsive use to the extent that taking the medication overrides other functions. The addict continues to use despite adverse consequences of a biological, psychological, social, and/or spiritual nature.

Just to confound things a little more is the fact that individuals respond differently to specific opiates due to individual genetic variations.

> *"An injection of Demerol makes me absolutely euphoric. I get that rush, throw up, and I am good to go for a couple of hours. But I have got to tell you, I had a whole box of morphine and that stuff did not work for me. I got so frustrated with it that I stomped the vials with my foot."* As related to me by a 32-year-old Emergency Department physician.

How Opiates Impact Multiple Organ Systems -Opiates act upon brain areas that regulate stress. Our stress response capability is blunted by opioids. That is why some addicts comment to me that opiates "take all my stress away." The body always seeks balance, so there is a price to pay for this "stress-reducing effect." The price is a "stress-producing effect." This opioid blunting of stress alters our stress response system to the point that we become overly sensitive to normal stress when the opiate is removed. This is one of the reasons opiate addicts complain of stress and anxiety during acute withdrawal. Unfortunately, this abnormal stress response may continue to occur for months to years after detox. This abnormal stress response is part of the Post Acute Withdrawal Syndrome discussed in detail later.

Recovering opiate addicts can also experience a condition called anhedonia which is the inability to experience pleasure from things that usually make people feel happy.

Akin to anhedonia but separate and distinct is a rebound depression that can be experienced when the drugs are gone.

Thinking ability can be adversely effected by opiates and such effects may take time to normalize. These include memory problems, decreased verbal function, distractibility, and visual spatial impairment. This type of impairment can show up as a decreased ability to give and/or take directions. Opiates can also impact distance and depth perception.

> *"I was cruising down the Interstate when it happened. I thought I had enough room to get over, but I ran right into the other car and bounced off him and hit the railing. I wasn't drinking. All I had was a couple of Roxies. I totaled my truck though."*
> Elton is in treatment at the behest of his attorney. His charges include possession of a Schedule II and drug paraphernalia. (He had a used syringe and dirty spoon in the truck when he wrecked.)

Opiate use often causes insomnia. Then again, who wants to sleep through a $100 opiate high? Opiates also cause the pupils to become very small as in "pinpoint" in size. This does not happen with Demerol. As a matter of fact, one of the reasons many healthcare professionals (doctors, nurses, etc.) use Demerol is for this very fact. They figure pinpoint pupils might telegraph to other healthcare professionals that they are taking opiates. Not so with Demerol. There is one little drawback though, high doses of Demerol can cause seizures. If you are a nurse seizing in the middle of the ICU, you are giving as a clue to others that you might have a problem.

Opiates decrease the body's ability to fight infections. As a matter of fact, opiates promote the growth of viruses such as Hepatitis C virus and Human Immunodeficiency Virus (HIV).

Some of the lesser-realized effects of opiates involve the endocrine system. These are important enough to spend a little time on. Opiates increase the hormone prolactin. Prolactin is named for its ability to cause milk production.

In the male opioid addict, this may mean the development of breast tissue which is a condition called gynecomastia.

In the female opioid addict, it may mean menstrual irregularities and cessation of ovulation. This in turn means the female opiate addict may not be able to get pregnant while using opiates excessively. Then when she gets sober, she begins ovulating and is fertile again. This can lead to some surprises.

> *"Yes, I had sex with my boyfriend when I went off pass. I have been at the sober house for two months and I had two months of treatment before that. But I did not think I could get pregnant. We have been sleeping together for years without any birth control and no problem."* Conversation with Lisa who came to my office for a stomach virus that was making her vomit. Pregnancy test was

positive.

Another less know fact is that opiates can lower your thyroid functions. You may have an elevated TSH (Thyroid Stimulating Hormone) on admission, and it may be normal when repeated a few weeks later. This is a reason I generally do not jump to prescribe thyroid hormones for an opiate addict with a low TSH.

O.P.I.A.D. (OPIAD) stands for Opioid-Induced Androgen Deficiency. Chronic use of opiates results in lowering of testosterone levels. Symptoms include decreased sex drive (libido), decreased energy, decreased endurance, decreased motivation, decreased sperm count, and grumpiness. Testosterone levels generally start to normalize after a week or so of abstinence. Some of my patients tell me it took a month or so to get their libido back.

Since the recovering male opiate addict may have an increase in sperm count as testosterone levels increase, he may be more fertile.

I strongly discourage "treatment romances" but if an ovulating recovering opiate addict has unprotected sex with a recovering male with a high sperm count, it does not take a genius to predict what can happen. Lisa's scenario (above) is not that unusual.

Opioid-Induced Bowel Dysfunction (OIBD): Opiate addicts also tend to have all sort of gastrointestinal problems such as indigestion or gastric reflux (GERD), constipation with hard, dry stools, nausea, vomiting, bloating, and cramping. It appears that your brain develops tolerance to the effects of opiates, but your bowel does not. Hence, the opiate user has chronic constipation as long as he or she is using opiates. This will generally resolve with detoxification, but it is important to drink adequate fluids and start a stool softener if constipation persists during detoxification.

Naltrexone for Opiate Dependency- As previously noted, naltrexone comes in a form you can take by mouth (trade names ReVia and Depade) and in an injectable form (trade name **Vivitrol**). It is an opiate antagonist. This simply means it blocks the effect of opiate receptors in your brain. In other words, if you inject, inhale, or swallow an opiate, the opiate has no effect.

Dosage for Oral Pill Form: The dosage for opiate dependency treatment is the same as that for alcohol dependency treatment. Generally, oral naltrexone is taken at a dose of 50 mg by mouth a day. There are other dosing regimens, but the most common and probably the best way to go is with the oral form.

There is no optimal length of time for taking naltrexone, but if it works, six months to a year seems reasonable. There may be a "carry over" beneficial effect for months after the drug is discontinued.

Dosage for Intramuscular Injection: The recommended dosage of injectable naltrexone (Vivitrol) is 380 mg injected into muscle tissue (that would be in the upper outer quadrant of your butt) every four weeks.

Adverse Side Effects: Liver damage is a concern with naltrexone albeit the injectable naltrexone is less prone to cause liver damage. There may be pain at the injection site with the naltrexone XR (Vivitrol). I insist that any addict I am going to inject with naltrexone XR has a complete understanding of the drug and its side effects. Of course, I do the same with oral naltrexone. Before injecting naltrexone, it may be a good idea to try an oral dose of naltrexone to make sure there are going to be no adverse reactions. The injection is going to last for about four weeks but the oral form can be stopped at any time and that's the end of it. There are other possible gastrointestinal side effects as well as effects on mood.

The rationale for naltrexone in opiate addiction is that even if you use opiates, you do not get high. Since one of the problems with addiction is that the circuit from the reasoning part of your brain is not in sync with the emotional or desire part of your brain, you tend to cave in if the stimulus to use is overwhelming. You're not thinking at that point; you are responding like one of Pavlov's dogs.

However, with naltrexone on board, if you cave and use, the opiates do not work. The "desire to use" part of your brain is dampened. This gives the reasoning part of your brain a chance to kick in and lets you remember the undesirable parts of addiction.

Let me give you a real world example. Perhaps something like this:

> *You got out of rehab two weeks ago only to find out that your girlfriend has hooked up with one of your "using friends." The common denominator of your relationship with her was "Roxies." Since boyfriend number two has managed to run out of money (and dope), here she is showing up on your doorstep. She is a MAJOR TRIGGER, and after a brief non-intimate sexual encounter, she tells you she is getting drug sick and needs opiates. It is decision time.*
>
> *Do you call your sponsor? Nope, he would tell you to get the hell out of there or come pick you up, and he probably would not be very nice about it.*
>
> *Do you call your parents? Hell no, they hate this*

girl and blame her for your addiction.

Do you call her parents? Definitely a no! Besides, you are not a rat (street pride and junkie thinking).

Are you thinking with your reasoning brain or your desire brain? Face it. You are being controlled by your desire brain.

At any rate, she is aching and pacing and crying and sweating, and her pupils are as big as saucers. Being the empathetic (or pathetic as the case may be) person you are, you make "the call" to a dealer and spend some of that rent money your parents gave you. Now you are back into the life that cost you "everything." But what the hell – you have the junkie girlfriend and you have the dope. Party time! You cram some Roxy up your nose. NOTHING! You cram some more. STILL NOTHING! Your "girlfriend" is definitely loaded so the dope is real. You shoot up with her rig even though only the demons of addiction know where she has been and with whom while you were in rehab. Damn – Nothing! It must be that damn naltrexone shot they gave you two weeks ago. It actually works. Hell, you may as well not use. You look around, think about what has transpired and take an inventory like they taught you in rehab. You are with a loaded woman who is so sick that she would sell her soul, let alone her body, for a thirty milligram tab. You have taken advantage of her addiction. She has taken advantage of your addiction. You do not know what you may have caught. You have blown the rent money. You were already thinking about hocking the TV or maybe even pimping her out. You have let everyone down. You are disgusted with yourself. The good news is that you are not high and can actually think. Naltrexone has bought you some time. As the sun breaks across the sky,

*you make that phone call - the right one - and get
your butt back into recovery and her to the
emergency room.*

Pros and Cons and Comments: We just saw that naltrexone is not a cure. Addict behaviors become hard wired with continued use. In the case above, we also saw that if you do use opiates, while naltrexone is in your system, you will not get high. This may "buy you some time" and give your rational circuits a chance to kick in and override your dysfunctional reward circuits.

Naltrexone also works as a deterrent to help you not use (or "pick up") in the first place. Why pick up opiates if they don't work? Several recovering addicts have told me they used opioids while on naltrexone just to see if the naltrexone would work. I do not condone the opiate self-challenge test for many reasons, but I am not surprised addicts test it out – they are addicts. Unfortunately, if you over amp on opioids trying to get over the naltrexone blockade, you can overdose. You might not get high, but you can get dead.

One of the weaknesses of naltrexone is that it will only stop an opiate high. It really doesn't do much for the other addictive drugs. (Alcohol being the exception.)

Naltrexone may dampen the alcohol high, but you can drink through that with a little dedication. Plus, there are always other drugs that naltrexone does not block like benzodiazepines, cocaine, methamphetamine, marijuana, "synthetic marijuana" and on and on.

If your drugs of choice are opiates and you are serious about recovery, naltrexone can help increase your chances of recovery as part of a comprehensive program with the goal of total abstinence from all mood-altering substances.

Naltrexone is not addictive. One other warning you need to heed is that if you are loaded up on opiates, do not take naltrexone. Naltrexone taken while loaded will cause an instant and prolonged opiate withdrawal syndrome. I know a couple of addicts who tried it. They only did it once.

There are some situations in which taking this drug is mandated by professional boards as sort of an insurance policy that the healthcare provider addict will not use. This mandate is not unheard of for recovering anesthesiologists or nurse anesthetists as part of their contract to return to work.

Naltrexone's impact on testosterone levels is of particular interest to male opiate addicts. Opiate addicts often have testosterone suppression. Being off the opiates would be expected to improve this. Naltrexone appears to augment or increase testosterone levels.

There is data to support the practice of taking oral Catapres (clonidine), while on naltrexone. This combination appears to provide an improvement in stress response capability, a decrease in craving, and a decrease in emotional negativity.

Buprenorphine for Opiate Detoxification and Maintenance-Buprenorphine is an opioid and is classified as a controlled, dangerous, addicting drug with a Schedule III designation by the Drug Enforcement Administration (DEA). Trade names for buprenorphine include Suboxone and Subutex. Another buprenorphine preparation recently approved by the FDA goes by the trade name Zubsolv.

Buprenorphine is a narcotic pain medication. The buprenorphine formulations mentioned above are approved by the FDA for the "maintenance treatment" of opioid dependency. Opioid Maintenance Treatment (OMT), also known as opioid replacement therapy (ORT), is just what it sounds like. ORT means I am prescribing a different opioid to the opioid addict with the intent of maintaining him on the replacement opioid, which in this case is buprenorphine. Sometimes this is referred to as opioid substitution treatment because we are substituting one opioid such as buprenorphine for an abused opioid such as heroin.

The first drug approved for ORT was methadone.

I personally cannot embrace the concept of putting an opiate addict on another opioid with the intent that he or she may be on it forever. There is plenty of controversy about buprenorphine maintenance which has spawned several lively discussions (arguments) with some of my colleagues about this very thing.

According to my patients, there are doctors who prescribe buprenorphine at the drop of a hat (or a dollar). These doctors promote and sell buprenorphine as if it is a wonder drug. They prescribe it rather freely in what my patients call "Suboxone Clinics." The addict grapevine is replete with the names of the easy doctors. Not surprisingly, my addicts have no respect for these types of doctors and use them as drug dealers. As an extra added attraction, my patients generally pay cash.

Since I am usually admitting these patients to detox, I do get a biased view of what is going on in the "subs" world. However, it is not uncommon for one of these patients to show up with prescriptions not only for Suboxone, but also with prescriptions for Xanax or Klonopin and Vyvanse or Adderall all of which are from the same prescriber. I am going to try and stay politically correct here and limit my comments to my opinion that this "combo pack" makes absolutely no clinical sense to me in treating an addictive brain disease.

Here is another sub pearl. My patients often sell or buy Suboxone at $20 per 8 mg hit on the streets. Many of them incorporate Suboxone into maintaining an active addiction to heroin or oxycodone. If heroin is not available for any particular reason, they buy some sub on the street to get them by until they can get back to their drug of choice. The idea here is that Suboxone will stop the opiate withdrawal until the heroin is available again. Here is what Arthur had to say when I asked him if he had ever taken Suboxone.

"Yeah, Doc, I have used subs. I got them from a sub clinic. The last time was when the whole family drove to Disney World. I knew I could not be shooting up in the car or the motel in front of everybody." He laughs. "That would not go over well. So anyway, I took subs to get through the vacation and got back on roxies as soon as I got home. Plus, I had some subs left so I sold them to get more roxies. I also took some benzos I got from that quack doctor."

In all fairness, I want to state that there are also doctors who prescribe buprenorphine appropriately as part of a real, ongoing, monitored, treatment process.

Here are my thoughts. Addiction is a biological brain disease caused by ingestion of mood-altering chemicals, in this case opiates. If the addictive brain is submerged into an opiate bath on a long term basis, it would seem plausible that the continued exposure of the addictive brain to the opiate would cause progression of the disease. I believe buprenorphine maintenance could do just that.

I consider buprenorphine to be a harm-reduction drug. In other words, the addict has come to the conclusion that he or she cannot get off opiates. Therefore, they give up trying and get on buprenorphine.

There are some legitimate advantages to ORT. For one thing, it is legal. It also reduces some high risk behaviors, like sticking an unsterile and/or shared needle into your veins. While buprenorphine maintenance is not cheap, it is usually less expensive than a $150-a-day Roxy or heroin addiction. Plus, you generally do not have to hock your TV set, (or more importantly my TV set), to get the money for ORT.

A significant limitation with Opioid Substitution Treatment is that although buprenorphine may block a heroin high, you can still get loaded with non-opiate mood-altering substances like alcohol, marijuana, Klonopin, or whatever. A particularly dangerous practice is taking a benzodiazepine, like Xanax, with buprenorphine as this can shut down the breathing center in your brain. It is call respiratory arrest.

Being able to use other mood-altering drugs, while taking buprenorphine, is one of the limitations of "treating" only one drug, especially with another similar drug. The drug is part of the addiction problem but the core problem is the addictive process and the addicted brain. There is always the danger of replacing one addictive drug with another addictive drug or behavior.

Another problem I encounter with buprenorphine-dependent patients is that the detoxification process after being on buprenorphine maintenance can be rough and prolonged.

Having said all that, I have the credentials and special narcotics number to prescribe buprenorphine, and I do prescribe it. Here is how I employ buprenorphine.

Short-Term Detoxification: I prescribe Subutex (buprenorphine) during inpatient opiate withdrawal for what I define as short-term detoxification from opiates.

Acute opiate withdrawal from the short-acting opiates generally takes five to ten days. A full-blown withdrawal syndrome can present with the following:

- Muscle aches all over but especially in the legs and back
- Restlessness
- Restless legs
- Sweats and chills
- Skin crawling with goose bumps (also known as piloerection)
- Anxiety
- Panic attacks
- Fatigue
- Stomach cramps
- Nausea, vomiting, and/or diarrhea
- Yawning
- Insomnia
- Craving
- Light sensitivity
- Runny nose
- Watery eyes

I rarely prescribe buprenorphine (Subutex) for over fourteen days in the acute inpatient detoxification setting. Of course, buprenorphine is not the only medication I prescribe for the opiate withdrawal syndrome (OWS). Baclofen helps with muscle aches and also has some anti-craving properties. Odansetrone (Zofran) is a good choice for nausea and vomiting; plus, in and of itself, it may alleviate some of the OWS symptoms. Clonidine (Catapres) is an antihypertensive medication that limits over activity of adrenalin. This is important because OWS is accompanied by an excess of adrenalin secretion which can cause panic, anxiety, sweating, and elevated heart rate. I also employ non-addicted sleep aids if needed.

Long-Term Detoxification with Buprenorphine: If an addict has failed multiple treatments for opiate addiction and cannot seem to stay clean for over a month or two, I will consider a longer term detoxification period of up to six months. This will be done on an outpatient basis. ORT is not my first line treatment by any means, and I will only consider ORT after all else has failed. Prior to initiating long-term detox with ORT, I will encourage the use of Vivitrol injections, but if that is not an option, long-term detoxification may be indicated. I have treated only a very few patients with this regimen.

This does not mean I am casually handing out Suboxone. It means you must commit to six months of ongoing group and individual therapy. You must have clean drug screens with the exception of buprenorphine. You must go to meetings. You must have a sponsor. You must agree to sit down with me and your therapist at the end of six months, or less, for a reassessment with the goal of getting off the ORT. Once we begin titrating off of the Suboxone you need to commit to at least six months of formalized aftercare. I prefer a year of aftercare.

Buprenorphine is an addictive and dangerous medication. I have concerns about long term use of ORT, and the effects ORT may have on organ systems and the immune system. Buprenorphine does decrease cognition (thinking), and in combination with things such as benzodiazepines, the cognitive effects are worse. I definitely advise against prescribing it to a person who works at job that is designated as safety sensitive. As far as my own personal safety goes, I would not want someone on buprenorphine ORT operating on me or my family. Nor would I want a person on ORT piloting the commercial airliner I just boarded.

Another reason I generally discourage long-term opiate

replacement is that my empirical clinical impression about ORT versus abstinence was recently affirmed by an original research article in the *Journal of Addiction Medicine.* *

In the opioid-free recovering person, the brain employs specific areas when confronted with a cue or temptation to use. For instance if Janet, a recovering heroin addict, finds a stash of heroin that she had hidden from herself prior to going into treatment, that is a major temptation (or cue) to use. Trust me on this, if she finds a bag of dope, the event is going to create an emotion. (I have been there.) The emotions of being confronted with a cue can vary from joy and excitement to fear and repulsion. These feelings mean certain areas of her brain are activated. One of those areas is the Anterior Cingulate Cortex, which we will call the ACC. The ACC evaluates and re-evaluates emotions and also helps regulate emotions. Needless to say, in active addiction she was having emotional dysregulation. Finding dope will create joy and excitement in the active addict.

Another part of her brain, the Inferior Frontal Gyrus, which we will call the IFG, also comes into play. Her trained and recovery-minded IFG will help inhibit unhealthy responses. Her IFG assesses the cue or temptation as a bad or negative thing to do because there will be an undesirable outcome. The interaction of the IFG and the ACC causes her to experience fear and repulsion at the thought of relapse. This in turn leads to risk avoidance (she does not use the drug). When she resists the cue to use and gets though a high-risk situation, her circuits are strengthened even more, and her self-efficacy improves. CBT and other therapeutic processes help develop these parts of the brain to resist relapse. We have previously discussed the need to build and strengthen healthy circuits to overcome dysfunctional (addictive) ones. This is a prime example.

"It was just like my therapist said. You have to play

the whole tape through and not just react."

Playing the tape through means her IFG is capable of thinking of the adverse impact of using heroin and helps inhibit the behavior of using. The ACC is able to evaluate and re-evaluate the emotion being felt as the data from the IFG flows into the ACC. The IFG did not just get that way. She did a lot of work in therapy to help normalize her IFG function so that she is able to evaluate the negative consequence of a behavior. Her brain is no longer just reacting, she is making proactive choices. As a matter of fact, if we track her brain activity when confronted with a cue to use, we will see that her IFG is very active. She is developing the tools to resist relapse.

Now let us take a look at the ORT brain. Same scenario, the guy on ORT finds a bag of dope. His IFG activity is lower than the abstinent recovering addict because he does not need to develop skills to resist temptation if his brain is already saturated with a "legal" opiate like buprenorphine or methadone. This, in my opinion, is a major problem with opiate maintenance. You do not build the circuits to resist cued behaviors because you do not need them as long as you are on opiate maintenance. However, what happens when you get off ORT? You have not developed the brain circuits or skills to resist using cues. Therefore, you are a high risk to resume opioid ingestion. This is one reason that the "logic" of ORT escapes me. How can you recover if you are taking drugs that do not allow you to develop the parts of your brain that allow you to recover? Not only that, what happens to your brain receptors as well as the rest of your body when you expose it to opiates non-stop?

If you want more information about this phenomenon, read this article in the *Journal of Addiction Medicine*, "Patterns of Brain Activation During Craving in Heroin Dependents Successfully Treated by Methadone Maintenance and

Abstinence-Based Treatments." Hassein Tabatabaei-Jafari, et. al., Volume, No. 2, March/April 2014.

What about just going "cold turkey"? -Going cold turkey from opiates will probably NOT kill you unless you have some underlying medical problems, but it CAN kill you. It is really not a smart option. Acute opiate withdrawal causes all sorts of chemical imbalances in your brain. It is like "brain chemicals gone wild." You can even give yourself panic attacks by doing this. You can also further impair your already impaired stress response system. Also, due to the nausea, vomiting, diarrhea, and lack of appetite, there is a risk of dehydration and associated electrolyte imbalances. Craving is worse during a cold turkey experience. If you try to "cold turkey" and end up going out and buying more dope to stop the withdrawal, you are back into a relapse cycle. When you fail at your own detox attempts, you actually reinforce the pathological circuits in your brain telling you that you cannot live without opiates. Cold turkey is for turkeys.

Kratom is another mood-altering plant alkaloid with opioid-like effects. It is found in the leaves of a south east Asian tree called Mitragina speciosa. It activates several opiate receptors in the brain and is an opioid agonist. It can be taken by mouth or smoked. I mention it for several reasons. First of all, more and more patients are telling me they have used it. These patients usually have opiates as their primary drug of dependency. Supposedly it has stimulant effects at lower doses and opioid-like effects at higher doses. Kratom is "legal" at this time, but it is considered a "Drug of Concern" by the Drug Enforcement Administration (DEA). The patients I have chatted with about it tell me it is a poor opiate substitute, but it does not show up on a drug screen unless you specifically test for it.

"Yeah. I tried it. It was OK. I would do it again if it happens to be around. But with heroin so easy to get, why use kratom?" Marvin, 24 year old opiate addict.

Kratom detox is very similar to any other opioid withdrawal syndrome. All the restlessness, muscle aches, anxiety, nausea, vomiting, diarrhea, light sensitivity, sweats, chills, agitation, and lethargy come with Kratom withdrawal. I treat it with the same medications used to treat any opioid withdrawal syndrome. It lasts about a week or so.

Krokodil, which is Russian for crocodile, is the street name for an impure form of desomorphine. It is "popular" in Russia because the ingredients for homemade krokodil are readily available there. I think codeine is available over the counter in Russia. It is used intravenously. Krokodil is somewhat renowned for its ability to make your skin rot off at the injection sites. If you inject it, your skin can get sort of gangrenous green so that it looks like crocodile skin. Krokodil may be finding its way into the USA. A few on my patients claimed to have used it. Who knows if they did or not? They do not know what they got, but one had a couple of seriously sclerosed (hardened) veins that were impressive. Given the side effect profile, I don't think it will be very popular. But, I could be wrong.

DRUGS OF ADDICTION
Benzodiazepines

Benzodiazepines are anxiolytics which means they reduce anxiety at least initially. Benzodiazepines are also called sedatives. These drugs act primarily by inhibiting some brain nerve cell functions. The net effect of benzodiazepines is to calm the brain. However, these drugs can also induce euphoria in certain people. Some official clinical indications or reasons for prescribing "benzos" are:

- Anxiety Disorders
- Panic Disorders
- Insomnia
- Muscle Spasms
- Seizure disorders
- Alcohol Withdrawal Syndromes

Practice guidelines support only short-term use of benzodiazepines. There is ample reason for this. For one thing, benzodiazepines are addictive substances, and this is a major problem. It's not just a problem in the USA. For example, in the Netherlands, the problem of long-term benzodiazepine use increased to the point that the whole country stopped health insurance reimbursement for these medications. That was back in 2009. The fact that insurance no longer paid for the benzodiazepines did not cause much change in use by the chronic users. It appears the chronic benzodiazepine users cannot or will not stop taking these "short-term" drugs.

Benzodiazepine use is also associated with increased risk of motor vehicle crashes. Another disturbing fact is that they increase the overall risk of death. Indeed, research indicates any sleep medication increases the risk of death as much as three times than that of the people who do not take sleep medications.

Abuse Potential appears to vary among the different benzodiazepines.

The most "abused" benzodiazepines:
- Xanax (alprazolam)
- Valium (diazepam)
- Klonopin (clonazepam)
- Ambien (zolpidem)

Intermediately abused:
- Ativan (Lorazepam)

The less abused benzodiazepines:
- Serax (oxazepam)
- Librium (chlordiazepoxide)

It is obvious from this list that not all benzodiazepines are created equally from an addictive potential.

Why are some benzos more addictive than others? To understand the degrees of addictiveness, we are going to have to divert our attention back to that dynamic three-pound organ that sits inside each of our skulls and is called the brain.

In order for a drug to get from your blood stream and into your brain, it must cross a barrier aptly named the "blood brain barrier." If a drug easily dissolves in fatty tissue, it is called lipophilic or "fat friendly." The degree of fat friendliness determines how hard or how easy it is for a drug to cross the blood brain barrier and get into the brain. Highly fat friendly drugs cross the barrier more easily and more quickly than those drugs that are less fat friendly. Also, the quickness with which a drug crosses the barrier equates to how immediate the concentration of the drug will be in the brain. Achieving an immediate high concentration of a mood-altering drug in the brain is often referred to in addiction jargon as "a rush."

Valium (diazepam) and Xanax (alprazolam) are very fat friendly and quickly cross over into the brain. This rapid onset may in part account for the higher abuse potential of these drugs. While Klonopin does not seem to share their degree of fat friendliness, it is a potent benzodiazepine that is also a popular agent of abuse among my patient clientele.

Obviously, any benzodiazepine can be addictive, but I have yet to see a "benzo addict" whose primary benzodiazepine of choice is Serax (oxazepam) or Librium (chlordiazepoxide). As a matter of fact, when I tell my detoxing Xanax addicts that I am going to prescribe Serax for detox, they usually do not know what it is. Even more telling is the fact that if they are unfortunate enough to go out and relapse after treatment, they do not seek out Serax on the street. They go for Xanax, Klonopin, or Valium. Still, that does not mean that Serax is not addicting. Individual differences exist in individual brains. You cannot completely predict or judge what effects a drug will have on one person by the effect that drug has on another person.

Ambien (zolpidem) is a sleep medication that can cause all sorts of problems such as sleep walking, sleep eating, sleep driving, and amnesia. I think one of Ambien's street names says it all, "Zombie." I advise anyone in recovery to stay away from this controlled drug. I refuse to prescribe it for anyone. It can cause hangovers and impairment for over eight hours after taking it. I have treated people who use Ambien as their primary drug of choice.

> *"I would use it (Ambien) to get through my shift. I could take up to eight a day. I hate going to work because my supervisor is such a bitch. I really don't remember a whole lot of what happened that day.*

They said I was impaired at work. They say I just stood over a patient and held the IV line like I was catatonic. They wanted a drug screen, but I refused and told them I quit and left. Then I hit a couple of parked cars on the way home. I really don't know much about that either. But the police showed up at my door and arrested me. I do remember that."

Janet – Registered Nurse

Detoxification Issues with Benzodiazepines - Detoxification from benzodiazepines can be complicated by the fact that one may experience a reemergence and/or magnification of an anxiety disorder for which the benzodiazepines may have been prescribed in the first place. It may be difficult to distinguish whether the anxiety is due to benzodiazepine withdrawal or if the anxiety was there all along and was just masked by the benzodiazepines, or it may be a combination of both. It is usually a combination of both.

Anxiety and panic attacks must be addressed as the detoxification process proceeds. Otherwise, the person may feel the overwhelming need to leave treatment against staff advice and subsequently relapse. The basics of benzodiazepine detoxification include stabilization with one of the less-abused benzodiazepines, like Serax or Librium, and close medical monitoring by supportive and knowledgeable health care providers. Once the patient is stabilized, a slow titration off of benzodiazepines as clinically tolerated in initiated. Adjunctive measures include relaxation techniques such as deep-breathing exercises, cognitive behavioral therapy, and non-addictive, anti-anxiety medications if indicated.

Just for clarity, I want to state that the patients I treat for benzodiazepine addiction are usually not taking therapeutic doses as prescribed by their doctor. Although, some are taking the amount prescribed, the amount is a hefty one. It is not uncommon for addicts to defend their benzodiazepine prescription by insisting they "need it and the doctor says so." For the record, if you are taking your Klonopin as prescribed but you are doing so on top of a bottle or two of wine a day, you are not within "therapeutic" range, and you are going to detox.

Benzodiazepine withdrawal is dangerous and can be fatal! Do not quit taking benzodiazepines cold turkey!

> "I ran out of Xanax, and I was broke so I could not get any, so I just decided to stay there at the house. I woke up on the floor. I think I had a seizure, but I decided not to tell my wife because I did not want her to know what I had been doing. Then she and the kids got home, and we were all sitting there at the dinner table, and it happened again. She called EMS, and the Emergency Room doctor told her it was a withdrawal seizure. I had a bunch of tests including a CAT scan and a shot of Ativan. She told me it about scared the kids to death. She told me I could not come home. I guess she's tired of all the lies and the money for drugs. I would be too if I was her. I lied and told her I had straightened up. She may leave me over this and take the kids. I really screwed up this time. Right now I'm sore all over, and I feel like I am about to crawl out of my skin. I take three to four "bars" a day, sometimes more. I have got to stop all this, Doc, or I am going to lose everything that is really important to me."
> Earl is a 27-year-old plant worker and father of three. He presents with shakes, sweats, elevated blood pressure, and elevated pulse rate. This is his first day of what will be a fourteen-day detox.

It is well known among the general population that seizures can occur during benzodiazepine withdrawal. Since there may be no warning, the consequences can be disastrous. For instance, a withdrawal seizure could occur while the person is driving a vehicle down the interstate. That has happened to several of my patients. I guess I need to qualify that statement. That is what several of my benzodiazepine-dependent patients told me they think happened prior to the motor vehicle crashes.

What is not as well known among folks, including benzodiazepine users, is that benzodiazepine withdrawal seizures can be recurrent and can progress to an uncontrolled state (status epilepticus) that can be life-threatening.

Benzodiazepine withdrawal can also result in a psychotic state with hallucinations and paranoia. This psychotic symptom as well as seizures can usually be avoided if the benzodiazepine addict is medically detoxified by capable professionals in a timely manner.

There is also evidence to support decreased cognitive functioning due to long-term benzodiazepine use may last for months after the drugs are stopped. It may take six months or longer for the cognitive effects to resolve. Morever, according to the National Academy of Neuropsychologist, there is concern that some of the cognitive defects due to chronic benzodiazepine use may be permanent.

DRUGS OF ADDICTION
Marijuana

Marijuana refers to the plant, Cannabis sativa. The main psychoactive ingredient of marijuana is THC (tetrahydrocannbinol) albeit there are others psychoactive alkaloids present. Indeed, THC is one of almost five hundred compounds found in the plant.

There are two cannabinoid receptors identified in humans that have been studied rather extensively, namely CB1 and CB2 receptors. Others may exist.

CB1 receptors are located in the brain and other parts of the body including the reproductive systems of females and males. As a matter of fact, men with a significant history of using marijuana are twice as likely to develop testicular cancer later in life.

The neuropsychological effects of THC are explained by the fact that THC acts on CB1 receptors located within the brain. Activation of these receptors results in activation of the brain reward system (mesolimbic dopamine system), and this causes the marijuana user to feel good. THC also suppresses "excitatory" nerve transmission which in turn decreases anxiety and promotes a feeling of relaxation (mellowing out). THC also has pain-relieving (analgesic) properties. Impaired motor function and impaired memory accompany intoxication. Interestingly, the stimulation of CB1 receptors by THC can result in a panic response in some individuals.

Cannabinoid brain receptors help control body weight and maintain nutrient/energy balance. This is one of the reasons marijuana use may cause an increased appetite (the munchies).

CB2 receptors are located primarily on immune tissues and in white blood cells (immune cells). They are also located in the brain. Marijuana's THC impacts the immune system. This may be both good and bad. An anti-inflammatory response may decrease pain, but an anti-inflammatory response may also increase cancer risk. Then again some investigators think there may actually be some anti-cancer protection from cannabinoids. If this sounds confusing, that is because it is. It is actually hard to get reliable data on the effects of smoking marijuana due to a host of confounding variables, not the least of which are ethical constraints connected to research parameters. It is known that marijuana smoke does contain some cancer-causing agents (carcinogens).

Marijuana use can decrease nausea. This anti-nausea or anti-emetic effect occurs through THC's action on CB2 receptors.

CB2 receptors are also involved in the perception of pain. This is true for acute as well as chronic pain. Indeed, research is targeting CB2 receptors for pain control, and several new agents targeting the cannabinoid receptors have been developed but not yet released for medical use. The ultimate goal of pharmacological relief of pain is to develop a medication that will stop the pain but not cause mood alteration.

Marinol (dronabinol) is pharmaceutical THC (Schedule III) used to stimulate appetite in anorexic AIDS patients and/or to combat nausea due to chemotherapy for cancer patients.

Cesamet (nabilon) is another legal (Schedule II) synthetic cannabinoid used primarily to treat nausea due to cancer chemotherapy. Due to all the side effects associated with nabilon, it is not a first choice medication for this particular indication.

Risks Associated with Marijuana Use: The risk for adverse effects is somewhat dependent upon when the person started using the drug. Recurrent use before the age of eighteen years old is associated with long-term brain damage. This is reflected as memory and attention problems as well as lower overall intelligence compared to nonusers. Marijuana users who do not start using until after eighteen years old do not manifest this type of brain damage, at least not to a significant extent.

So what does this mean in the real world? It means that the early onset marijuana smokers have less of an IQ at thirty-eight years old than they had as kids. To use the vernacular, they got less smart. If you are less than eighteen years old when you start smoking dope and have an IQ that is average (50th percentile) and you keep smoking dope, by thirty-eight your IQ will drop to below average. Your marijuana addiction will have you "dumbed down."

It seems the bottom line here is that if you want to settle for less of a life, smoke dope as a teenager.

Marijuana Psychosis: If you show up at the emergency room with a psychosis after smoking marijuana, your future outlook is disturbing, and your risk for developing schizophrenia or an ongoing psychosis is very high. It is actually as high as seventy percent.

There is some predictive vulnerability to getting lasting adverse effects from marijuana use. This means we can figure out who is at risk for some really bad consequences if they smoke dope. The risk for brain damage increases if you are a younger person, and if you use a lot. The risk for developing an ongoing psychosis is primarily found in users with a high genetic risk for developing schizophrenia. If you are genetically loaded for schizophrenia, marijuana may push you over the edge and activate the disease. Marijuana use is what science refers to as an independent risk factor.

This risk factor for activating a chronic mental illness can be avoided.

Addictive Potential: Tolerance to the effects of marijuana does develop with chronic use, and there is a marijuana withdrawal syndrome. For some reason, females tend to become addicted to marijuana faster than males. I have treated many addicts whose primary drug of choice is marijuana. Historically, they often started using in their early teens. They use compulsively despite continued adverse consequences. They are addicts. They generally smoke throughout the day. Subsequently, when they stop using, they often have withdrawal signs and symptoms and subsequently resume marijuana use to ward off those uncomfortable feelings.

In chronic marijuana users, there is a predictable marijuana withdrawal syndrome. Valarie's situation is a good example of what to look for in marijuana withdrawal:

> Valarie was admitted to treatment two days after an arrest for possession of marijuana and paraphernalia. *"I really need something for my nerves right now. I feel like I'm going to have an anxiety attack. Look at my hands. I am shaking and I am sweating. I never sweat. Plus the nurse was a real bitch to me [irritability]. Can I get something to help me sleep [insomnia]? Like, I have not slept in two days but who sleeps in jail? Right? For that matter who eats in jail [poor appetite]? That is probably why I have such a headache right now. Can you give me something for that? I will tell you this, if I did not have all this legal crap on my head I would be using right now [craving]."*

> Valarie has the full marijuana withdrawal spectrum: anxiety, mild tremor, sweating, sleeplessness, decreased appetite, craving, and

irritability. This is no surprise if you know that she smokes marijuana all day, every day and has done so for years. Her irritability may escalate into outright aggression in another day or so. She may act out by cursing, slamming doors, or "getting up in someone's face." Actual physical violence would not be the norm, but when this particular withdrawal symptom kicks in, she will be at risk for leaving treatment and relapsing.

Marijuana withdrawal can compound withdrawal from other drugs such as opiates. Another clinical pearl about marijuana withdrawal is that Wellbutrin (bupropion) can make it worse. Marijuana withdrawal usually peaks in the first week or so of abstinence but may persist in milder form for four weeks or so.

Addicts and Marijuana: Even if marijuana is not the drug of choice for an individual addict, marijuana can certainly lead him or her back into their drug of choice.

"I know, I know." She said in a whiny voice. *"I had six months sobriety, and everything was going good, and everyone was proud of me. One evening, I just decided to smoke a joint with some friends I happened to meet up with. I did it and nothing bad happened, so I did it again and again. Then one of them showed up with some heroin, and I just could not resist. Of course, by this time I had stopped going to meetings because I had used pot and did not want to be a hypocrite, and I stayed away from my sponsor because she would kick my ass. She would have made me pick up a desire chip, and I could not bear that*

embarrassment. I screwed up, huh?"
Brenda – 27-year-old heroin addict in
the middle of a child custody battle.

<u>Gabapentin</u> (trade name Neurontin) is actually an
anticonvulsant used to treat seizure disorders. However, it
appears to have some usefulness for addicts at several levels.
This medication is also approved for the treatment of some
types of chronic pain and for Restless Leg Syndrome (RLS).

Gabapentin appears to be beneficial in the treatment of the
marijuana withdrawal syndrome. As noted above,
marijuana withdrawal is relatively prolonged. The ongoing
withdrawal symptoms promote the marijuana addict to
relapse. Gabapentin taken from day one of stopping
marijuana and continued as needed may double the addict's
chances of stopping the drug altogether.

One study published in 2012, showed that gabapentin eased
marijuana withdrawal symptoms, reduced craving, and
improved thinking (neurocognitive executive functioning).

In my addictionology practice, I have pretty good success
prescribing gabapentin for patients who report marijuana as
their drug of choice. Gabapentin can be effective in
decreasing the anxiety and aggressiveness related to
marijuana withdrawal. It also helps these addicts stay in
treatment. I start it as soon as the person has signs and
symptoms of detox. I generally prescribe 100 to 300 mg four
times a day for a week or so, and then I gradually reduce the
dosage on a weekly basis based upon the patient's response.
As a very general rule, I usually continue prescribing the
gabapentin for at least thirty days. If there are co-occurring
problems that have responded to gabapentin (such as
anxiety), I may continue it as long as needed.

DRUGS OF ADDICTION
Herbal Marijuana Alternatives (HMAs)
Synthetic Marijuana

Let us start from the beginning by quoting John W. Huffman, the professor of organic chemistry who first made these now ubiquitous synthetic cannabinoids. When asked about using synthetic marijuana, he said that people who use this stuff are "idiots."

Herbal Marijuana Alternatives (HMAs) were initially synthesized as part of the noble quest to develop medications to treat symptoms of multiple sclerosis, for anorexia associated with AIDS, and for an adjunct to help combat side effects of chemotherapy. Unfortunately, but not totally unexpectedly, the HMAs got hijacked for their abuse potential and became popular with the "drug crowd" rather rapidly. "Spice" was a popular name for HMAs for a while, but this gave way to the rather inclusive term of "synthetic marijuana."

One of the alleged reasons for their popularity among marijuana users was that HMAs were not detected on routine drug screens. Indeed, fifty percent of marijuana users have tried HMAs.

These drugs are bad news. The drug is sprayed on some type of dried vegetable substance, such as herbs or spices, and this serves a smokable vehicle to get the drug into the smoker's brain. HMAs act on the same receptors as the THC in marijuana but in a different manner. They are as much as five hundred times more potent than regular marijuana. This is not a good thing. Marijuana's THC does not fully occupy the CB1 receptor (THC is a partial agonist), but HMAs occupy one hundred percent of the receptor (full agonists). This means among other things that tolerance to HMAs develops rather rapidly, and there is an increased risk of addiction.

There are other differences but the bottom line is that HMAs can cause anxiety, paranoia, agitation, and psychosis. Indeed, HMA withdrawal can cause severe anxiety and depression. Furthermore, the use of HMAs by mom as early as two weeks into a pregnancy can cause severe birth defects.

A HMA-induced psychotic state can last from five days to five months. It may even trigger a person who is genetically susceptible to mental illness into a life-long psychotic illness.

One of the problems with determining all the health consequences of HMAs is that there are currently four major chemical groups called HMAs, and there are variations constantly occurring within these groups. You never really know what you are getting when you use a HMA. The only thing you can be sure of is that you are getting and using substances that are neurotoxic. I recently had a patient tell me he was smoking "homemade synthetic." Neither he nor I have any idea what was in it, but according to him, it was making the rug crawl out from under us as we sat in my office. He had not used for over two weeks.

You also never really know what the stuff is going to do to your other body systems and body organs.

> *Casper, Wyoming, March 2012. After smoking some synthetic weed with the packaged name, "Blueberry Spice", several young people started to have nausea and stomach pain. For three people, the symptoms continued to get worse and they experienced the loss of the ability to control motor movements or even stand up. Three young people were diagnosed with kidney failure. A dozen or so more got sick, and a total of six were hospitalized. Some of these young people did not know each*

*other, and the only thing they had in common was
the use of Blueberry Spice.*

Most of the people whom I evaluate who are using this "stuff" are younger, as in late teens to mid-twenties. Many of them tell me that since they began using synthetics, they do not get the same high from marijuana anymore, so they stopped using the "real marijuana."

Since synthetics are a "moving target" in that the psychoactive components vary and change, it is hard to really keep up with them. Parents are often confused as to what to look for even if they suspect their child is using HMAs. Even though the particular HMA compound may not be identified, they all tend to exhibit similar effects.

The acute physical signs that may accompany HMA use include:
- Elevated heart rate
- Elevated blood pressure
- Blood shot eyes (injected sclera)
- Dry mouth (xerostomia)
- Nausea with or without vomiting
- Warm skin and possible temperature elevation
- Sweating
- Jerking muscle movement
- Seizures, rare but can occur
- Kidney failure is rare but has occurred
- Electrolyte imbalance
- Physical effects that last up to 8 hours or so after using a HMA.

Of particular concern is the possibility that these physical effects may culminate in a condition called rhabdomyolysis. Rhabdomyolysis is the syndrome that occurs when muscle tissue is damaged to the extent that the muscle cells essentially dissolve (lysis). The muscle protein (myoglobin) gets into the circulation and overloads the kidneys to the extent that they stop working (kidney failure). Muscle jerking cited above can be a warning sign that rhabdomyolysis might occur. Prolonged seizures can also cause it.

Rhabdomyolysis results in muscle damage and kidney failure that can disrupt the balance of electrolytes in the body and cause heart rhythm problems. The treatment is to stop the toxic drug and correct the electrolyte imbalance.

While we're on the subject, I want to interject that HMAs are not the only abused drugs that can cause this condition.

The psychological effects of HMA use may include:
- Relaxation
- Mood elevation
- Anxiety
- Panic attacks
- Paranoia
- Hallucinations
- Suicidal thoughts

Withdrawal from HMAs is similar to that seen with marijuana, only worse.
- Restlessness and agitation are quite common
- Irritability to the point of "going off" on others
- Nausea
- Vomiting
- Decreased appetite
- Muscle cramps
- Muscle twitches
- Tremor or mild shakes
- Insomnia

Gabapentin is useful medication for treating an HMA Withdrawal Syndrome. Here is a clinical example of how effective it can be.

Douglas is two days into cold turkey withdrawal from "legal weed." He uses as much as he can get, and he uses all day long. He has used it this way since it became available. He went from marijuana to synthetic in order to dodge the drug screens at work.

"I just do not feel right, dude. Like I almost went off on my roommate over nothing. I mean like I almost slugged the guy. And I am not a violent person. Everyone is just getting on my nerves around here. And it is like I need to work out or something, man. Like I need to stretch my muscles. I am sweating and jumping out of my skin, man. People tell me to calm down but screw that! I cannot calm down! And I am not sleeping, and when I do doze off, I get these crazy dreams. I am thinking about blowing out of here and just saying screw the job and the judge and everybody else. You have got to help me here, Doc."

Doug is exhibiting signs and symptoms of acute HMA withdrawal. He was started on gabapentin 300 mg by mouth four times day for detox. This is what Doug reports the next day.

"That medication really helped me slow down. It is like I can actually think. I'm still irritable, but it is better. Nowhere like it was. I was able to sit in group and not feel like running out. The sweats are better too. That crap [HMA] was really on top of me. I heard it could be bad, but that stuff was making me crazy. So, how long do I need to stay on this medication, Doc.?"

Doug is asking a very good question. There are no approved protocols for HMA detoxification that I know of. As with marijuana withdrawal, I start with gabapentin 100 mg to 300 mg by mouth four times a day. The first week is usually the roughest time for detox. As Doug said, it is a high risk time to "blow out" of treatment. Depending upon the patient's clinical response, I taper the dose schedule down to three times a day for week. If all goes well, I then go to twice a day for a week and then once at night for a week. The patient needs monitoring as I judge the dose and duration of treatment by clinical response. I have some HMA recovering addicts who elected to stay on a reduced dose of gabapentin for several months with beneficial results. Some have reported to me that when they got off the medication "too early," they had anxiety, irritability, and craving.

Since HMAs are neurotoxic, it comes as no surprise that HMAs can lower your seizure threshold. That means you are more prone to having a seizure if you use them. From a clinical perspective, this means that if you are "poly-addicted" to say alcohol or Xanax and you also smoke HMAs, you are at a greater risk for seizures during acute withdrawal. Gabapentin, being an anticonvulsant, offers some protection against seizures.

As previously noted, gabapentin is effective in treating the thinking difficulties experienced by some marijuana addicts, and I believe it also helps improve cognition in HMA addicts. My experience has been that HMA addicts tend to have trouble encoding information for weeks after the last use of HMAs. Until the person can start to encode information, he cannot get maximum benefit from treatment. As a result, these patients often require longer term therapy.

Of special note is that if your drugs of choice are alcohol plus marijuana and/or "synthetic marijuana", gabapentin might be worth a try to decrease post-acute withdrawal symptoms and craving. It's pretty much uncharted territory, but there is a clinical and medical rationale for giving it a try. At any rate, if this applies to your situation, I am open to discussing it with you.

As for "synthetic marijuana" …

"You have got to be an idiot to use this stuff."

DRUGS OF ADDICTION
Hallucinogens

Hallucinogens were quite "the craze" during the sixties. LSD (Lysergic Acid Diethylamide) was popularized by the "Flower Children" of the era, but it had already been around a while. Mescaline (peyote) enjoyed a brief reign of popularity but that soon tapered off. Then came the ever present "magic mushrooms" (psilocybin) and mushroom tea.

PCP or Angel Dust is a nasty drug characterized by coma, convulsions, catatonia, and combativeness. It peaked relatively rapidly and then went away. Well, it sort of went away. There are still a few "mini-pockets" of use in the USA, and there is an ever-present fear that it may return as a fad drug again.

Ecstasy or XTC is MDMA (3, 4-Methylenedioxy-methamphetamine). It gained popularity in the Rave era and pushed LSD down a notch or two in popularity. Its latest street name is "Molly," and it is pushed as pure MDMA. Many of my younger patients have tried it, but its use is rarely cited by them as a regular occurrence or as a drug of choice. The hallucinogen scene is currently being inundated with a new crop of synthetic hallucinogens, so you never really know what's in the latest street version.

I've decided not to delve into the seemingly endless esoteric quagmire of the classification and sub-classification of hallucinogens. However, I will ask you for one indulgence concerning terminology. When I use the term psychedelic drug, I am referring to the "classical hallucinogens" which are primarily LSD, LSD-like substances (Morning Glory seeds, etc.), psilocybin, and mescaline.

Overall, there is little indication that these classical

psychedelic drugs cause long-term mental illness. However, for the record, there are individual casualties related to psychedelic drug use. Predisposed persons who use psychedelics may trigger a prolonged psychosis. Moreover, psychedelic use can become compulsive in nature. "Bad trips" or "recreational misadventures" can result in dangerous and/or fatal behaviors. It is also reasonable to anticipate that people who use LSD will try other drugs. Overall, LSD and the LSD-like psychedelics appear to be less harmful than some other illicit drugs, but they are far from being harmless. I do not condone the use of these psychedelics, and as Schedule I drugs, they are all illegal.

The term "hallucinogen" is somewhat of a catchall term that can be rather misleading. The various "hallucinogens" floating about generally cause perceptual distortions and mood alterations but overt hallucinations are not the norm or the goal of ingestion. The typical hallucinogen or psychedelic user, if there is such a person, usually tells me the goal is entheogenic (spiritual) or to attain "mind expansion" and a mystical type experience.

The risks associated with some of the "newer" substances such as "meow meow" (a synthetic cathinone similar to Ecstasy found in "bath salts") is yet to be determined. Given the chemical structures of these drugs, I anticipate all sorts of pathological brain changes replete with mood disorders and thinking impairments.

Indeed, some hallucinogens are known to cause appreciable brain damage. There is ample evidence that ecstasy causes significant damage at the chemical communication spaces between nerve cells (synapses). Ecstasy or MDMA is referred to as a "hallucinogenic amphetamine" and as an emphathogen. An emphathogen purportedly causes one to feel empathy, love, and emotional closeness. I guess that means if my twenty-three-year-old son ever starts hugging me and telling me how much he loves me, he's going for a drug test.

Unfortunately, XTC might also cause him to have rapid heart rate with the possibility of a heart arrhythmia, a stroke, severely elevated temperature, muscle damage, kidney damage, and of course brain damage to the areas of his brain that control emotions. The most common mood problem I would anticipate him developing would be depression. I would also be fearful that his substance-induced mood problem might be a long-term effect. There is one more problematic variable. The odds on his getting pure uncontaminated ecstasy are just about zero.

From a clinical perspective, it has been my experience that hallucinogen addicts are something of a "different breed." Maybe people who gravitate toward hallucinogens are a preselect group, or maybe the hallucinogens change them. It is a "chicken or egg" thing. I am not being judgmental here, just saying. Some of these addicts even refer to themselves as "psychonauts." In all fairness, I want to note that these patients are mostly into "synthetic hallucinogens" and rarely limit use to just that. I also want to note that other patients in the treatment center, those who do not use hallucinogens, may put forth unsolicited comments about them such as, "That dude is really strange, Doc."

I've treated several patients who cite their drugs of choice as hallucinogens, and many consider themselves very versed in hallucinogenic and psychedelic psychopharmacology. They tend to wax on about the beneficial nature of the drug and its benign effects while sitting right there on my exam table in a treatment center. Again, let me emphasize we do not know what short and/or long term damage some of these new hallucinogens may wreak upon the human brain or the human body.

Here are a couple of things that we do know.

> Law enforcement authorities in Minnesota reported the death on March 16, 2011, of a 19-year-old male, and the hospitalization of 10 others between the ages of 16 and 21, caused by the use of a synthetic hallucinogen, 2C-E, a phenethylamine.

> A single drop of a "new" synthetic hallucinogenic" into the nose of a 21-year-old male caused him to seizure and die at Voodoo Fest 2012 in New Orleans. It was a "free dose." The drug is called N Bomb or 25i, and several other deaths throughout the USA have been attributed directly to its use.

Ketamine or Special K is a dissociative anesthetic that can not only alter perceptions in the user, but can also cause that person to have an out-of-body experience. Ketamine is a legal, Schedule III controlled drug used in surgery as an anesthetic. It is used to put you into a controlled coma during the surgical procedure. It follows that ketamine abuse could put the user into a helpless state making him or her totally vulnerable to sexual assault or whatever other atrocities might be dealt out at the hands of whomever.

The urban story of the Ketamine user who wakes up with a fresh surgical incision on his flank may have little credence, but it does illustrate the street lore surrounding how helpless the drug can make you. Then again, you only need one kidney, right?

Ketamine is not meant for chronic use. What kind of idiot patient would want to stay in a dissociated semi-comatose or comatose state?

That would, of course, be my kind of patient.

In such a patient I might find significant impairment in thinking ability or cognition. I may actually note cognitive problems even in infrequent users. Ketamine users tend to have memory problems of various sorts including short term memory. *"Did I turn the bath water off?"*

These brain effects may present a picture similar to dementia. With heavy users, there may be delusions and dissociative feelings. *"It's like I'm looking down at myself doing things."* These patients also tend to be depressed.

There is a school of thought that Ketamine addicts are trying to escape life in general. I will leave all that theorizing to the therapists. What I know is that ketamine abuse can damage you.

Dextromethorphan (DXM) in high doses can have effects similar to those of the dissociative anesthetic ketamine. Therefore, I have elected to include it under the heading of hallucinogens. DXM is found in Robitussin DM cough syrup. Robotripping is the act of drinking large amounts of Robitussin DM with the intent of experiencing stimulation, euphoria, depersonalization, distortions and/or hallucinations. The observable effects of acute intoxication include stumbling or staggering about, nausea, vomiting, high blood pressure, high heart rate, and confusion.

There are genetic differences that influence the different effects of DXM on an individual. For example, a person who is genetically loaded to be "an extensive metabolizer" will have greater euphoric effects from DXM. On the other hand, a low metabolizer who uses the drug will be prone to develop DXM toxicity which could result in a medical emergency such as a coma.

Medicinal uses of Hallucinogens: An increasing number of scientists are investigating the therapeutic uses of different hallucinogens for treatment of a variety of psychiatric and medical conditions. For example, ketamine may ultimately have a place in the treatment of some types of depression. Topical ketamine may help with certain types of chronic pain.

LSD research has resurfaced as an adjunctive (add on) medication for alcoholism in some circles. This doesn't mean we will be handing out LSD take-home doses at the treatment center.

LSD is classified as a Schedule I drug and is therefore illegal except in controlled research settings. It is an historic fact that Bill Wilson, co-founder of Alcoholics Anonymous, did take LSD under supervision in what was considered therapeutic doses. He reportedly considered it to have some value for treatment of alcoholism, but that it was by no means curative.

Clearly, the people I treat aren't exactly taking therapeutic doses of anything. Indeed, when it comes to hallucinogens, they may not even know what they are getting from the dealer because not even the dealer knows what is in some of that stuff, and contaminants abound.

Detoxification from Hallucinogens: There really is no detoxification per se as there is no identified withdrawal syndrome. The addict may undergo rebound depression and visual disturbances, but most psychonauts are aware of the cause and rarely disturbed by their presence. Flashbacks are generally recognized as just that, a flash, which passes within a short time. It is not unusual to see this type of addict sort of "zone out" at times.

Persistent Flashbacks: There is an uncommon residual consequence from hallucinogen use known as the Hallucinogen Persisting Perception Disorder. HPPD is a re-experience of the hallucinogenic experience while not using the hallucinogen. In order to be considered a disorder, this expereince must be distressing to the individual. There is some concern that specific types of antidepressant medications may trigger this condition. I have not treated a person with HPPD, yet.

DRUGS OF ADDICTION
Amphetamines
Methamphetamines
Amphetamine Type Stimulants

A Brief History: Amphetamine compounds have been around since 1887. In the early 1930s, amphetamine was available as an over-the-counter nasal inhaler. Of course, some people quickly figured out you could remove the contents from the inhaler and eat the strips, or better yet soak them in your coffee.

Then during the mid-thirties, amphetamine was commercially popularized by the pharmaceutical companies as an antidepressant for the treatment of "mild depression." The practice caught on rapidly. During World War II the American and British pilots used amphetamines while their German counterparts used methamphetamines (meth). Supposedly, Adolph Hitler himself was no stranger to meth.

The Japanese also handed meth out to soldiers, workers, and pilots, including the kamikaze types. After the war, Japan was plagued with a meth epidemic supposedly due to easy access, secondary to huge methamphetamine drug stockpiles.

Interestingly, although the popular opinion was that amphetamines were innocuous, the medical literature of those days describes amphetamine abuse and psychotic reactions due to such abuse. Evidently, this literature was dismissed, overlooked, or simply dwarfed by an avalanche of advertising from the pharmaceutical companies. (Sound familiar?)

By the 1960's an iatrogenic (caused by doctors) amphetamine epidemic was in full swing in the United States. Indeed,

President John F. Kennedy was treated with amphetamines by Dr. Max Jacobson. Dr. Jacobson was also known as "Dr. Feelgood" as well as "Miracle Max." Max made thirty-four visits to the White House to treat the president, and he even accompanied JFK to the Vienna Summit in 1961. "Miracle Max" supposedly treated lots of other celebrities before losing his medical license, but to my knowledge none of them except JFK had access to nuclear weapons.

As the adverse effects of pharmaceutical amphetamines became more apparent, the prescription use of the drugs declined. Unfortunately, as legal amphetamines became less available, the manufacture of illicit methamphetamines ushered us into a meth epidemic. The meth epidemic started in the 1960s and gained real traction by the 1980s. Various illegal methods are employed to make meth. Some are more hazardous than others. Consequently, "lab" explosions abound. It seems that every meth addict I treat thinks he or she has a connection with a cooker who makes pure meth, or they may have their own method for making the dope.

Amphetamines are stimulants that can be taken by mouth, sucked up into your nose, smoked, or shot into your veins. Amphetamines not only cause a surge or excessive release of two neurotransmitters (norepinephrine and dopamine) in your brain but also prevent your brain from taking them back up into storage as it normally would. This results in a higher than normal concentration of these chemicals in the communication spaces (synapses) between brain cells in certain areas of your brain. This internal imbalance causes subjective and objective effects.

The desired subjective effects are:
- Euphoria ("I feel great!")
- Wakefulness ("I could drive all night and then some.")
- Alertness ("I can really study on this stuff.")

- Energy ("Can I work a triple shift today?")
- No hunger ("I don't even think about food... or water.")
- Increased self-confidence ("I'm good with dogs. He won't bite me.")
- Increased physical endurance ("I'm amping up to run this 10K.")
- Perceived increased coordination ("Watch this skateboard trick!")
- Increased strength ("I amp up to lift weights. But I get headaches too.")

The objective or observable effects include:
- Elevated heart rate
- Irregular heart rate (at times)
- Heart attack (usually in older persons)
- Elevated blood pressure
- Stroke (uncommon but possible)
- Increase rate of breathing
- Enlarged pupils
- Dry mouth and nose
- Sweating
- Elevated temperature
- Shakes (usually mild)
- Seizures (with high doses)

Amphetamine Psychosis is characterized by paranoia, persecutory delusions (*"The CIA is after me"*), auditory and visual hallucinations, thought reading (*"They are reading my thoughts"*), and anxiety. When I was coroner of East Baton Rouge Parish back in the early 2000's, it was not unusual to encounter meth addicts with this type of psychosis.

For those readers who do not live in Louisiana, an explanation is in order. In Louisiana, the coroner not only investigates death, he or she also does commitments to mental institutions for those who are dangerous to self, dangerous to others, gravely disabled, and unwilling or unable to seek voluntary help.

If you are amped up on methamphetamine and duct taping your window blinds shut and wrapping aluminum foil around your head so that the DEA agents in your ceiling crawlspace cannot control your thoughts, you might be experiencing an amphetamine psychosis. You will definitely come to the attention of the authorities if you start shooting holes in your ceiling to ward the agents off. You will also end up being committed by the coroner to an acute psychiatric ward. You will stay there until you clear up, and that may take a couple of weeks. Fortunately, most users do not escalate to this level of drug-induced insanity.

The paranoia that can be associated with excessive methamphetamine intake does offer a "teachable moment." Therefore, I will pass on this survival tip. If you are lost on the rural back roads of Louisiana and come upon a house trailer with aluminum foil all over the windows and a pair of tennis shoes dangling by their laces from the power line out front, it is best if you do not stop there to ask for directions. You might even want to speed up a bit just in case the "cook" inside is about to make a mistake and blow the place, and you, off the map.

Most methamphetamine addicts I know get on a "run" and go until the point of exhaustion. They generally acknowledge getting paranoid as part of the package. Then they pop a few Xanax or whatever and crash for a day or so.

Research indicates that there may be a genetic link between vulnerability to an amphetamine psychosis and schizophrenia. This is especially interesting from a clinical perspective because it appears that antipsychotic medications may protect against some of the neurotoxic effects of amphetamines.

Therefore, if you come in to my treatment center paranoid and over-amped due to an amphetamine or methamphetamine psychosis, we may be able to modulate some of the brain damage you are having by prescribing an antipsychotic medication to you. The importance of this is underscored by the fact that up to twenty-five percent of meth addicts who experience a drug-induced psychotic episode develop a prolonged or even permanent psychotic disorder.

Meth Mouth: Why does smoking methamphetamine cause your teeth to rot? There are several reasons including dry mouth, grinding your teeth, constriction of the blood vessels that keep your teeth nourished and alive, poor hygiene, cigarette smoking, and poor nutrition. What did you expect, pearly whites?

Meth Skin: I can walk through the mall and pick out the meth addicts. They are usually skinny, have a leathery-looking skin with lots of skin sores that they often try to hide with makeup and long sleeves. By the way, the camouflage is not working.

They are suffering from compulsive skin picking due to meth which may ultimately leave them with plenty of scars as reminders of their meth addiction. Just for the record, not everyone who has a compulsive skin picking disorder is a meth addict.

Meth addicts also tend to have what is known on the street as that "premature aging thing." They really do appear to be aging rapidly. I think it's a combination of malnutrition, osteoporosis, loss of teeth, generally poor hygiene, multiple bouts of various infections (skin infections, pneumonia, sexually transmitted diseases), trauma from being in high-risk situations, muscle wasting, lack of medical care, lack of follow up with medical care, and brain damage.

Meth Brain: Methamphetamine addiction causes brain damage. That damage results in impaired ability to correctly interpret facial cues or expressions.

For instance, let us say that you have been off methamphetamine for a few days, and you are famished, so you drop into a McDonald's for a Happy Meal or two. The young lady at the counter smiles and asks, "Can I help you sir?" You misinterpret her facial expression of pleasantry as one of disdain. You in turn scowl and quip, "What the hell is your problem, bitch." She thinks you're crazy and so does the cop eating his Big Mac at the table behind you.

Okay. It may not be that overt, but if you misinterpret facial communications, people will find you weird, uncaring, or just detached. For example, if your fiancé is experiencing a great deal of emotional pain and it is written all over his face and you ignore it by asking what time the Circle K closes tonight, you are not going to have much of a bonding experience. If you cannot build a concept of the other person, you certainly cannot establish a realistic relationship with that person. Plus, the meth brain may not be able to control aggression and/or stupid outbursts. Needless to say, all this creates social awkwardness if not ostracism. This is really bad news for your recovery because much of recovery is built upon establishing healthy relationships and social recovery networks.

Another meth brain effect is called anhedonia or the inability to experience pleasure. This tends to improve with abstinence but takes time and interaction with others. Yet another added attraction of methamphetamine addiction is the fact that you may magnify negative feelings and be more sensitive to pain.

Long-term effects of meth are dose and time related. The longer and more you use, the more chance you have for long-term brain damage such as dementia and even an increased risk for Parkinsonism.

Medications for Meth Brain: There are no specific medications to treat amphetamine dependency however, Wellbutrin (Bupropion) may help with cognitive functioning and may decrease craving. Remeron (mertazepine) may also be helpful in reducing cravings. Use of either of these antidepressants for amphetamine craving alone would be an "off label" use.

Ibudilast is an asthma medication that has been used in Japan and South Korea for about twenty years. It is not currently available in the United States but human clinical trials are underway in the USA to determine if this is a safe and effective drug for the treatment of methamphetamine addiction. Here is the reason it might work. When a meth addict stops taking meth, there may be ongoing brain inflammation with resultant damage and/or death to some types of brain cells. Ibudilast may stop this process which would mean less brain damage and improved ability to think and subsequently to be involved in an addiction recovery process. It also means the addict will feel better and subsequently have less craving. There is also data to support the use of ibudilast in opiate withdrawal and even in pain management.

Meth Withdrawal Syndrome: There are no specific medications for amphetamine withdrawal. There is a rebound or crash state most people refer to as a detox or withdrawal phase. My patients usually arrive in a crash state and look like they have been shot out of a cannon. They are lethargic, and the number one concern is getting to sleep. Once we assess them to rule out any acute medical issues that need attention, I generally let them sleep or crash for however long it takes. Upon awakening they are usually pretty hungry and in need of some attention to personal hygiene. Their moods usually range from dysphoric to anhedonic initially, but anxiety and depression can also be present. This acute phase lasts for about a week. Needless to say, major fatigue is often a part of the withdrawal process as is craving.

DRUGS OF ADDICTION
Cocaine

Cocaine has been around a long time. If you were an Inca roaming about the Andes Mountains 5000 years ago, you were probably chewing on a cocaine leaf to keep you going.

Cocaine was medicinalized for the treatment of mental illness in the 1800s by its most famous proponent Dr. Sigmund Freud, who used it himself for many years. He extolled its virtues, wrote a book about it, and even tried to cure one of his morphinist (morphine addicted) colleagues of his opiate addiction by turning him into a cocaine addict, or cocainist. That did not work out well. The poor guy became psychotic behind the cocaine use. Things got so bad that his family and other colleagues were glad when he went back to being a plain old, garden variety morphinist. To my knowledge, Freud's dramatic therapeutic misadventure (failure) is the first medically-documented attempt to treat an addiction to one drug with another addictive drug. Unfortunately, Freud was not the last to make such a flawed medical judgment.

Cocaine use reached "fad drug" heights in the 1970s. Some of us remember the golden razor blades worn on gold chains around the necks of cocaine users, and let's not forget the snorting spoon charms, etc. The route of administration was to snort it up the nose. In addition to being a stimulant, cocaine is also a local anesthetic or numbing agent that constricts blood vessels. You constrict those vessels enough, and the tissue will die. That's why I saw many a perforated nasal septum in those days. I would just look into the nose, and there would be no septum. The patient would usually just shrug his or her shoulders like it was no big deal. I tended to not ask about other mucous membranes.

The fad drug status declined, but the use did not. Addicts

are still smoking and shooting cocaine, but from what I have seen, intranasal use (snorting) has declined. Regrettably, I have witnessed a resurgence of IV drug users who combine cocaine with heroin. This especially dangerous combination is called speedball.

Then there was crack! Crack became popular in the mid-1980s and is still with us. Crack is a solid, smokable form of cocaine. When the crack rock is heated, it makes a cracking sound, hence its name. Most of the addicts I see who give their drug of choice as cocaine nowadays are crack addicts.

Cocaine is a powerful stimulant with properties similar yet distinct from amphetamines. It is shorter-acting than amphetamines which means a cocaine psychosis is shorter than an amphetamine psychosis. The shorter-acting property of cocaine also means you have to keep using more often to keep "high." The rush may last only five to ten minutes with residual effects hanging around for an hour or two. Cocaine activates the reward system in the brain, changes circuits, and causes addiction. Women tend to progress more rapidly than men into cocaine addiction.

Short-term effects include:
- Euphoria (Which is the reason for using it.)
- Feeling alert and wakeful
- Increased energy
- Anxiety and restlessness (Therefore alcohol is ingested to knock the edge off.)
- Paranoia
- Psychosis
- Dilated pupils
- Elevated heart rate (risk of heart attack)
- Elevated blood pressure (risk of stroke)
- Sweating and elevated body temperature
- Sexual dysfunction (impotency)
- Seizures

Longer term effects:

- Enlargement of the left side of the heart (Left Ventricular Hypertrophy) can occur with chronic use and predispose the person to heart attacks and sudden cardiac death.
- Psychosis
- Generalized deterioration of brain function can give a clinical picture of early onset dementia with chronic use. We have already noted that cocaine causes blood vessels in the body to constrict or clamp down. The blood vessels in the brain are no exception. Within two minutes after cocaine use, those vessels are constricting and cutting the blood supply to nerve cells. That can mean a seventy percent reduction in the amount of blood going to those brain cells, and with repeated use, it gets worse. If your brain cell is deprived of oxygen, it can die (neuronal death). Needless to say, this leads to more major life problems as it is difficult to make rational decisions with dead brain cells.

  I have noticed over the years that there are few older cocaine addicts around. I am not aware of the exact reason(s) behind this observation. I do not know if they just die young or experience brain burn out, or end up in jail. Whatever the reason this observation supports the notion that cocaine is not a forgiving drug.

Cocaethylene forms in the liver when alcohol is taken into the body while using cocaine. As noted above, some cocaine addicts drink alcohol to take the edge off. This actually intensifies the euphoric effect of cocaine and makes it last longer. Unfortunately for the addict, cocaethylene is more toxic to the heart and brain than either substance used alone.

Medical Treatment of Cocaine Addiction:

Disulfiram (Antabuse) which is discussed under the section for alcohol dependency treatment may help decrease cocaine use in cocaine addicts. This only works for some cocaine addicts who have a certain genetic makeup.

Baclofen has been associated with longer involvement in treatment, decreased craving, and decrease drug use in cocaine addicts.

An anti-cocaine vaccine is being developed and is supposed to go into human testing in 2014. The idea is that the vaccine attaches to the cocaine molecule and stops it from getting into the brain. We've discussed the blood brain barrier before. Even if we had the vaccine, it would not be a "stand alone" treatment for cocaine addiction. Booster vaccinations would be required. Addiction therapy would also be needed to maintain motivation and compliance.

Withdrawal: Cocaine withdrawal is similar to meth withdrawal. Expect fatigue, depression, anhedonia, and of course craving. That's right, craving.

> You just woke up in a treatment center. You have been kicked out of the house. You spent all your money. You hocked your grandmother's wedding ring. You missed a court ordered drug screen some dealer has your (soon to be ex-) wife's car. You stink, you need a bath. You have no idea how you got that hickey on your neck or elsewhere, and in the back of your addict brain is one predominant thought, *"I could sure use a hit of cocaine right now."*

Given all the consequences you are currently facing, you will probably choose to stay in treatment, at least for a while, and hopefully you can decide if you have had enough of the drug life yet. Do not expect that craving thought just to go away. That will probably be with you a long, long time.

DRUGS OF ADDICTION
Cigarette Tobacco

I am going to focus on cigarette smoking as the addiction of reference here rather than nicotine alone as the addiction. The two are not interchangeable. If cigarette smoking was just nicotine addiction, I could slap a nicotine patch on you, and that would solve the problem. It doesn't! Who really knows what the 4,000 other chemicals are doing to your brain? I do not, but I do know that a chemical called acetaldehyde appears to be involved in this addiction process. As with all addictions, the younger you are when you start smoking cigarettes, the worse your addiction will become.

Cigarette smoking is directly responsible for cardiac disease, blood vessel diseases, chronic obstructive lung disease (COPD), lung cancer, and a host of other cancers. The list goes on and includes risks of second-hand and third-hand smoke. I am going to limit my discussion to the addictive nature of cigarette smoking. To that end, here are some pertinent facts that cigarette smokers need know.

- Alcohol drinking increases cigarette smoking behavior.

- Cigarette smokers who are addicted to opiates smoke more than non-addicted smokers.

- Smokers require more opiates that non-smokers to control acute pain.

- People with chronic pain hurt more if they smoke cigarettes.

- Cigarette smokers have more pain after an operation, and they do not heal as fast. This is true for all tissues including bone healing. Of course it is. If you are trying to heal a broken bone or a skin graft, or whatever, the last thing you need to do is cut off the blood supply by twenty-five percent, make your platelets sticky enough to block even more blood supply, flood the wound with carbon monoxide, and top it all off with a hydrogen cyanide bath! Knowing this, if you are wondering why a non-smoker has a bone heal rate of ninety-five percent, and your cigarette smoke poisoned bone has a heal rate of only sixty-eight percent and takes longer to heal, you probably won't get an invitation to join the local Mensa Club.

- Cigarette smokers have a higher rate for an "unsatisfactory" face lift. (See above.)

- Cigarette nicotine withdrawal and detoxification are rougher if you are a drinker.

- Alcoholics are more likely to have depression during cigarette smoking withdrawal.

- Quitting or even cutting down smoking is associated with a better chance for recovering from other addictions.

- There is a genetic risk factor, which if you have it, tends to make recovery from cigarette smoking harder.

- Sleep problems are associated with smoking over a pack a day. Many smokers are "light sleepers." Cigarette smoking-induced sleep problems include not only taking longer to get to sleep but also waking up more during the night as well.

- Menthol reduces your lungs' defenses that try to keep the poisonous, chemical laden smoke out of your airways. By blocking your natural defenses, menthol promotes increases in the concentration of toxins in your blood, brain, and other organs when you smoke. In short, menthol lets you smoke more and harm yourself more.

Cigarette smoking addiction is a primary, chronic, progressive, and destructive brain disease that destroys your body's organs and organ systems.

Acute detoxification from cigarette nicotine takes about six to twelve weeks. Yep, that is right. If you are addicted to a pack a day, your brain receptors will physically scream for nicotine and cigarettes for up to three months. That is how long it will take your brain receptors to downsize to a "normal" number.

Of course, the number of receptors is not the only factor that encourages smoking and relapse. You have trained your brain that cigarette smoking has positive effects such as decreasing anxiety and elevating your mood. This is the "brain circuit" part of addiction.

When you decide to stop cigarette smoking, there are specific brain regions that you call upon when you are resisting the temptation to smoke. When you activate these brain regions you <u>focus attention</u> upon not smoking; you strive for <u>emotional control;</u> you initiate <u>decision-making</u> processes, and you deal with the <u>conflict </u>of wanting to smoke but knowing it is bad for you and yours.

As it turns out, bupropion (Wellbutrin, Zyban) activates these same brain processes and this may be how it helps addicts recover from cigarette smoking addiction. Bupropion may decrease weight gain and negative mood states associated with cigarette smoking cessation.

If you and your healthcare provider decide on using bupropion, it is best to start taking it a week or two before you plan to stop smoking. The reason for this is that it may take that long to get the maximum effect of the medication.

Nicotine Replacement Therapy (NRT) helps with cigarette smoking addiction recovery. The best results with NRT appear to come with using a combination of the nicotine patch and nicotine lozenges or nicotine gum.

Nicotine patches start with the 21 mg patch each day for up to six weeks, then drop the dosage to the 14 mg patch for a couple of weeks, then use a 7-mg patch daily for two weeks to finish the detox off.

Lozenges come in 4 mg and 2 mg sizes. If you smoke within thirty minutes of waking up, go straight to the 4 mg. Use a lozenge every one to two hours as needed for the first six weeks, then use a decreasing dosage schedule to wean yourself off them at week twelve.

Nicotine gum comes in 2 mg and 4 mg. If you are at a pack a day, go to the 4 mg. Chew one piece every one to two hours for up to six weeks, then drop to one every two to four hours for a couple of weeks and finish up with one every four to eight hours for two weeks.

You can become addicted to the gum.

Combination therapy: Nicotine replacement (patches, lozenges, gum) can be combined with bupropion (Zyban, Wellbutrin).

Nortriptyline (Pamelar, Aventyl) is an antidepressant that may double the chances for smoking cessation. It would be an off label use but is worth consideration if other treatments fail.

Varenicline (Chantix) is a drug that partially stimulates nicotine receptors while it blocks nicotine from smoking cigarettes. It may find use in the treatment of other addictions, but some of the side effects are worrisome. These include mood swings, bad dreams, violent behavior, heart problems (even in people without heart disease), suicidal thoughts, suicidal behavior, suicide, depression, blackouts, and/or psychosis. Obviously, given all these possible side effects, any person on Chantix requires adequate monitoring.

Chantix is banned for airline pilots and air traffic controllers. France has pulled Chantix from the government formulary due to its side effects.

More than Meds: In addition to medication, there are other things you can do to stop smoking. It is best to plan a stop date, enlist support from others, and consider some behavioral techniques. It is also a good idea to have some "competing thoughts" and "competing behaviors" as part of your armamentarium.

Women become "more addicted" than men. Hormones, especially progesterone, increase the power of craving when a female is exposed to a using trigger. Women have a better chance of quitting if they start at the end of a menstrual cycle. Of particular significance is the fact that middle-aged female smokers experience more decline in their thinking ability that non-smokers.

What about auriculotherapy? Auriculotherapy is stimulation

or acupuncture on the ear. There is no scientific data to support any benefit from this process.

Myth Busting: It is absolutely **not true** that you should wait until you "get over" your other addictions to stop smoking. The cigarette smokers' standard defense when I encourage them to address their cigarette addiction at the same time as some other dependency is:

> "One thing at a time, Doc. I plan to stop as soon as I get over this [insert primary drug of choice here] addiction."

If you expect me to agree with you, you are dead wrong.

Continuing your smoking addiction is addiction. People who stop smoking have a better chance of not returning to their other "drugs of choice." This means that people who do smoke are more prone to relapsing back into their other drugs of choice. Excuses are excuses and part of the addicts' defenses to keep using. Bill W. died of cigarette smoking addiction! Hopefully the current cigarette addicts reading this will not choose such a death as their legacy?

DRUGS OF ADDICTION – INHALANTS

Nitrous oxide (NO2) also called "laughing gas," has been around a couple of hundred years. Indeed, it is used as an anesthetic for some dental procedures. Interestingly, according to the American Dental Association, five percent of the dentists who develop addiction problems report self-use of NO2.

In my patient population, NO2 is rarely the primary drug of dependency. I have treated only three NO2 addicts in my entire career. The "desired" effects described by these patients included euphoria, mellowing out, floating outside my body. Actually, some of the effects sounded similar to those experienced with ketamine. NO2 does activate the reward system of the central nervous system.

Nitrous oxide is readily available and easily obtained because it is the gas present in "whippets" Whippets are metal vials of compressed food grade NO2 that are used as cartridges in reusable whip cream dispensers. There are also dedicated devices or drug paraphernalia that can be used to fill a balloon with NO2 from the compressed vials. The idea is to fill the balloon up and inhale NO2 from the balloon.

Prolonged use of nitrous oxide can cause vitamin B12 deficiency. One consequence of B12 deficiency is nerve damage. This nerve damage can show up as numbness in the hands and feet and is called peripheral neuropathy. Muscle spasms of arms and legs may occur also. Another sign of a low B12 level is enlargement of one's red blood cells, a condition called macrocytosis. In rare cases, nitrous oxide can cause psychosis and/or delirium. Prolonged use can also cause dark blotches, or hyperpigmentation, to develop on the skin.

Another possible adverse effect is brain damage due to

decrease oxygen to the brain. If your lungs are full of NO2 and no O2, you might be killing off brain cells.

NO2 use in pregnant females can cause birth defects. Indeed, there is concern that passive exposure to female staff members in a dental office setting that uses NO2 as an anesthetic may have adverse reproductive effects including miscarriage.

Diagnosis of NO2 dependency can be difficult if the addict does not acknowledge usage. However, there are two blood tests that can become abnormal with repeated NO2usage. They are homocysteine and methylmalonic acid.

Treatment for neurological damage caused by NO2 is intramuscular injections of vitamin B12. Recovery does not occur overnight but it generally does occur, for the most part. The NO2 addict may have some residual damage that could be permanent.

Dust Off refers to compressed gas used to blow dust off computer keyboards and such. It is not just compressed air. Dust Off's Material Safety Data Sheet lists difluroethane as a toxic ingredient. Adverse effects include heart rhythm disturbances, unconsciousness, and death. Frostbite is another hazard.

Since the Dust Off high lasts only a minute or so, the user must continuously inhale the substance in order to maintain the high. Users tell me they tend to pass out, wake up, and use again. Besides giving users a nudge to the reward centers, this method of use sensitizes the heart to rhythm problems and decreases oxygen to the brain and other vital organs.

If you are wondering, why in the world anyone would

inhale Dust Off, you might want to go back to the section on adolescent substance use. One inhalant addict I treated told me he used Dust Off because it doesn't show up on a drug screen. He's right; as a matter of fact, he could be dead right. I had one adult, who almost died from using Dust Off, give me this reason for his near death experience.

> "I was detoxing from the pain pills again, and I felt like crap. I had no money and no car and was thinking about who I might be able to call for some dope when I saw the can of Dust Off. I heard it could give you a buzz or even an opiate high. So, I said what the hell and gave it try. I woke up in the emergency room with a hell of a headache because I hit my head when I went out. The last thing I remember before waking up was tightness in my chest and then I felt a big hard thump. It was like my heart was going to explode." Arnold, 27-year-old opioid addict.

The huffer or Inhalant abuser has a wide variety and readily available number of neurotoxic inhalants to choose from. Inhalants are literally everywhere. Huffers are usually in their preteens or early teens. If they live, they tend to move on to other substances as they age. Inhalants of choice include gasoline, paint thinner, solvents, spray paints and whatever happens to be available. The desired effects are to attain an alcohol-like intoxication. Toluene does activate the brain's reward pathways, but it also does a lot of other things. Toluene inhalation is associated with sudden sniffing deaths, liver injury, kidney injury, and/or permanent brain injury.

Huffer kids are usually pretty easy to spot. For one thing, they frequently smell like solvents. Physically, they may have runny noses, irritated eyes, and a rash about their lips and noses. If they are into paint huffing, they may have paint on their fingers and/or under their fingernails. Psychologically and socially, they tend to have mood swings, may be depressed, and do poorly in school. Huffers are often loners.

AN OVERVEIW OF DETOXIFICATION

Some people live in a chronic state of detox. It IS a horrible place to be, and in keeping with the insidious onset characteristic of addiction, you may not even know it IS happening to you. By definition, the person experiencing chronic detox is physiologically dependent on some type of mood-altering substance. His or her brain has been saturated with mood-altering toxic chemicals so long that the brain, by necessity, has made adaptive changes to function.

One of the changes is that the brain's reward system has been physiologically and psychologically conditioned to view using the drugs of dependency as necessary for survival. The drug becomes the first consideration for any and all decisions and activities. The world is constricted around the drug, and the addict's life is revolving around obtaining the drug and taking it.

As we previously discussed, the brain, in the presence of a mood-altering chemical, will seek balance or homeostasis. For instance, if your brain is immersed in a sedative, your brain will gear up its activity to counteract the sedation. This neurological reaction has clinical implications for prescribing addictive drugs such as benzodiazepines and others. For purposes of illustration, we will use benzodiazepines as our example.

If you have anxiety, Xanax may help you in the short term. However, as time goes on, the Xanax may cause or worsen your anxiety. This can occur in as short a time as two weeks. Here is why that can happen:

1. Xanax works by suppressing brain function.

2. This brain function suppression triggers your brain to seek balance by increasing brain activity.

3. As the benzodiazepine wears off, your brain which has increased its activity, is now in an overly activated state. That state is anxiety. In other words, as the Xanax wears off, you get anxiety from the Xanax rebound. This is called drug withdrawal. In short, you are detoxing.

4. This withdrawal anxiety prompts you to take the benzodiazepine to suppress your withdrawal symptoms.

5. This in turn triggers your brain to continue to adjust to the sedative drug by gearing up with more activity.

6. After a short while, your brain develops tolerance to the drug, and you feel the need to increase the dose or to boost the drug effect by taking an additional drug, such as Ambien or alcohol.

7. This will help dampen the detox cycle your brain is now caught up in but only for a limited time. The cycle tends to get worse and reinforces itself.

8. In addition to all this going on, you are experiencing cognitive slowing which is one of the side effects of benzodiazepines and benzodiazepine-like drugs.

9. To combat that slowed thinking, you might end up on an amphetamine like Adderall.

10. This of course may increase the need for more benzodiazepines.

11. This is the epitome of a "vicious cycle."

This neurochemical balancing act is why prescribing benzodiazepines for a long period of time can cause dependency. This can create a neurochemical mess.

"If I run out of my Xanax, I am in trouble. I ran out two days ago, and I could not get a hold of my doctor to call a script in because it was the weekend, and I do not have any refills left. I could not get to sleep last night, so I drank some red wine and that helped, but I was a nervous wreck this morning so I was not sure if I should take my Adderall or not. I was aggravated with the kids because they were in slow motion and almost missed the bus. I must have yelled at them ten times to get them going. Then I got to work and had a horrible morning. Our first patient, Mrs. Morgan, got on my nerves more than usual. I got so upset with her complaining that my blood pressure was up, and I was sweating and almost had a panic attack. I even got shaky. Thank God, Sally takes Xanax, and she gave me a couple of hers until I could get a script from Dr. Willwrite. I think I will get him to increase my dose, so I do not run out again. I need my Xanax and I cannot function without it because of my anxiety gets out of control." Margie is a 37-year-old single parent in charge of billing and diagnostic coding for a physical therapy clinic. She started on Xanax to get through her "nasty" divorce. She has been on Xanax for two years with increasing doses and is now prescribed 2 mg three times a day. She is also on Adderall 30 mg a day for adult onset Attention Deficit Hyperactive Disorder "diagnosed" one year ago. Margie is essentially sleepwalking through life in a chronic state of sedation versus drug withdrawal and has a brain that is trying to compensate for the chemical mess it is floating in. At this point, the chronic Xanax

withdrawal may be amplifying or even causing
the symptoms she took it for in the first place.

Margie's new diagnosis of adult onset ADHD and her subsequent "need" for prescription amphetamines are worth reassessing. She was a quiet child in grammar school and high school, got good grades, and went on to become an accountant, all without any signs of ADHD. Yet, one year ago while under a great deal of stress and taking a benzodiazepine, she was having some concentration issues and was diagnosed with ADHD based solely upon those symptoms. In her words, "I never really took any test for ADHD. He just asked me a few questions, and it [Adderall] really helps me get my work done."

If Maggie decides to get off all this Xanax, she needs to do so in a controlled and monitored manner. If she just decides to stop it, she will experience a dangerous acute detoxification syndrome.

Acute Detoxification Syndromes refer to the predictable and sometimes unpredictable signs and symptoms that occur due to the abrupt discontinuation of a mood-altering chemical that has caused a pathological adaptation by the brain.

I often tell my patients to envision the brain as a big coil or spring. If a spring is left to its own accord, it will have no stress on it and will just sit there in a state of balance.

If I grasp each end of the spring and stretch it out, that is the equivalent of your putting a stimulant into your brain. When I let go, that is equivalent to your no longer putting the stimulant into your brain. The spring bounces back but not to its normal state initially. It goes to a compressed state first. That compression is the equivalent of the rebound depression seen during amphetamine and cocaine detox.

If I grasp each end of the spring and push the ends together as far as I can, that is the equivalent of your putting a sedative into your brain. When I let go, that is equivalent to your no longer putting the sedative into your brain. The spring bounces back but not to its normal state initially. It goes to an overextended state first. That overextension is the equivalent of the rebound anxiety seen in alcohol and/or benzodiazepine detox.

In both scenarios, the brain, like the spring, will finally reach a "resting" state (homeostasis), but that new steady state may be different from the original resting state due to the wear and tear on the spring.

For every action, there is an equal and opposite reaction. If you drink alcohol or take benzodiazepines, you are suppressing brain functions. When you stop drinking or sedating, the brain rebounds with hyperexcitability. That is called detox. This presents as anxiety, sweats, shakes, high blood pressure, high pulse rate, insomnia, nausea, vomiting, diarrhea, agitation, aggression, seizures, psychosis, delirium, and/or death in severe cases.

If you are addicted to amphetamine, methamphetamine, and/or cocaine, you are artificially increasing your brain functions. When you stop eating, smoking, snorting, or shooting the substance, the brain rebounds with decreased activity. This presents as fatigue, depression, anhedonia, emotional numbness, slowed thinking processes, and need for prolonged sleep.

The specifics of detoxification for the various addictive drugs were discussed under the headings of the individual drugs. Unfortunately, there are few purist addicts. By that I mean the heroin addict may also take benzodiazepines and/or smoke marijuana and/or smoke cigarettes and/or drink alcohol. You do not just detox from one of these; you detox from all of them. I must admit this can be somewhat challenging at times to both the patient and the medical staff.

Another confounding variable occurs when you ask the addicted person how much they are using. This is called the self-report, and it may be flawed.

Police officers commonly get inaccurate self-reports: *"I only had two beers, occifer."*

You might think that would not be the case in a detox center, but it often is. Actually, many times the addict does not know how much he or she has been drinking or using. There are lots of reasons for this. The point here is that initial self-reports on the amount of alcohol and other drugs being consumed are often not accurate. Some patients minimize the use of substances and others maximize their use.

Why would you minimize? Well, you may not know how much you use, especially if you are having black-outs or nod outs. You may want your record to show you don't have a problem or that you don't use illegal drugs or that you don't want your parent or wife or judge to know what you use. The fact that your record is protected by HIPPA is of little solace if you are in this mindset.

Why would you maximize? One reason to overstate your usage is to gain "street credit" or for "junkie pride" as we used to call it. Sounds dumb, but we are talking about an impaired brain here. The other reason would be to maximize the amount of detox medication you can get. We call this "drug seeking." Medically, we do not rely solely upon the patients' reports of discomfort during detox. We monitor for signs of detoxification and treat accordingly. If you're loaded on detox medications, you are not detoxing. I do not believe there is any clinical benefit from a painful detox. Actually, I believe just the opposite, but there will obviously be some discomfort.

Then there is the addict who brings drugs into the treatment center or gets somebody else to drop them off. These folks can get very creative. The big question here is not how they do it but why they do it. I have discussed it with enough of those individuals to have some insight into their reasons.

The obvious reason is that he or she is an addict and that is what addicts do. They make sure they have a ready drug supply. Forget logic as you know it. This person is thinking with an addicted brain. It comes as no surprise to me that as soon as Zolie got to the treatment center she ran into the visitor's bathroom and hid a bottle of Xanax in there and gobbled a few down "just in case" she started detoxing. That actually sounds pretty normal to me. That is why we search visitor's bathrooms on a regular basis.

Another motive for bringing drugs into treatment is "the defiant gesture." Zolie may be attempting to show everyone, including other patients, just how bad she is. This type of addict is steeped in the druggie culture and may be looking for some street credit by this behavior. She may be so afraid of failure that she is testing us to see if we do find the drugs. If we find them, the patient may feel she is in a safe place that will keep drugs out. If we do not find her stashed drugs, she has outsmarted us and has little respect for the program and even less faith that it will work. Remember we are dealing with an addictive and impaired thought process here. If there is a strong sense of recovery in the patient community, the other patients will not tolerate this. By bringing drugs in, the addict endangers everyone else's sobriety also.

Another reason might be due to a lack of trust. We tend to judge others by ourselves. If I cannot trust myself to make it to the store with enough money to buy diapers for my baby, how in the world can I trust you to detox me right? I cannot. Sure, you tell me detox will be okay, but I don't trust any of that BS. Therefore, the "logical" thing for me to do is bring in enough drugs to get me by during detox.

Then there is the antisocial narcissistic person who brings drugs in as part of a game to see if we can catch him. He may also plan to sell the drugs or use them for currency on other addicts.

There is a lot more to detoxification than just handing out medications. Each person requires a physical and mental assessment. Some patients have illnesses that compound risks associated with detoxification. A sixty-five-year-old alcoholic with chronic obstructive pulmonary disease and heart disease due to cigarette addiction is a lot different than a twenty-four-year-old alcoholic who works off shore and binge drinks when he is home.

The detox environment is also important. The attitude of the staff is extremely important. I don't need nurses who are punitive, but I do not need nurses who are pushovers either. Detox is a special area and requires special skills. My first encounter with "the iron hand in a velvet glove" nurse occurred when I decided to skip group since I was day two into a cold turkey detox. (That's how they did it in those days.) The short version is that I went to group. Her name was Miriam, and I am still grateful to her for how she helped me get through a very tough time.

POST-ACUTE WITHDRAWAL SYNDROME

Even in the midst of my addiction, I remained an avid reader. My reading was centered on emergency medicine which was a newly expanding field at the time. The more I studied, the more complicated those medical articles got. I mean that stuff was really getting hard for me to fully grasp. After about six months of sobriety, I realized it was not that the journals got harder, it was that my brain got softer. That realization was so disturbing that I was mortified with fear. How much had I lost? How much could I get back? After about eighteen months, I felt that I had gotten most of my brain function back. I even underwent a battery of neuropsychological testing to make sure I was not fooling myself into just thinking I was better. I learned in treatment that my disease had made me a master at self-delusion. Thankfully, I did well on the tests.

At eighteen months it was as if my peripheral vision had increased and the proverbial scales had begun to fall from my eyes.

It may take an addicted brain a couple of years of sobriety to recover. For that matter, there is empirical data that shows it may take five years. Obviously, some damage may never heal, but you can develop compensatory brain functions to help make up for any drug-induced defects.

Before we start talking about two to five years of sobriety, we need to concentrate on the initial weeks to months after acute detox. This is the period during which you may experience a condition called the Post-Acute Withdrawal Syndrome or PAWS.

If you are in early recovery, understanding this phenomenon is essential for you. Therefore, we need to explore this process not only so you can understand it, but also because there are some things you can do to mitigate or lessen PAWS. So, what exactly is PAWS?

PAWS is a time of physiological rebound and a time of early healing. I think one of the harshest symptoms of PAWS is anhedonia. If you cannot feel anything, you may just decide not to bother with recovery. Many of the patients I treat for relapse tell me the trigger was boredom. However, when we explore this boredom a little deeper, we often encounter emotional numbness or anhedonia. This lack of emotion is just one of the symptoms you can experience during PAWS; there are plenty more. These symptoms get better, and your brain and normal emotions will come to life, if you let them. Have hope because this too shall pass.

Opiate addicts often use opiates for energy. They use in the morning just to get out of bed and get going. Fatigue is one of their main PAWS complaints and a major relapse trigger. This improves with time and sobriety. Fatigue may also be a symptom of depression. If this is the case, there are certain antidepressants that target fatigue and are "more energizing" than others. Sleep hygiene also helps.

I have had patients come to me after a month or more of sobriety and tell me they feel like they are going through an acute detox again. *"I cannot sleep. I am on edge. I feel like I am crawling out of my skin. I have diarrhea. I get the sweats."* This is not acute detox: it is often simply being overwhelmed by life on life's terms. It may mean you are taking on too much and trying to fix everything you screwed up during your active addiction. Your brain and therefore your thinking abilities are still healing, and your reward receptors are still raw. Neurological, social, psychological, and even spiritual recovery is a process. To facilitate that process you must be working an active recovery program. That is one of the reasons a ninety-day primary treatment experience is needed to get on the road to recovery. There is a custom in Alcoholic Anonymous to tell the newcomer to attend ninety meetings in ninety days. I am not sure where that came from, but it certainly fits the research.

Most people who are coming out of an acute withdrawal are mentally clouded for a while. They have problems encoding new data (memory), and this is one reason the therapeutic messages in early recovery are often repetitive and redundant. Hence, we have another appropriate recovery slogan "Keep It Simple Stupid."

When you wake up in a new world, one without drugs and artificial emotions, you might feel overwhelmed. Anxiety, panic, irritability and feelings of generalized discomfort often follow. You may have a decreased ability to deal with stress, and subsequently little things rapidly become big things. You may overreact at times.

You may get bored easily. If your life has been centered around and constricted by addiction, you may not know what else to do or with whom to do it. You must give up pathological people, places, and things. You know it is the right thing to do, but it is not as easy as it sounds. Loss breeds grief, and addicts have a lot to grieve about. Sure, you are glad to be sober, but you may miss "the life" and all the hoopla that goes with it. Addictive drugs takeover reward centers and "love centers," and there is a real grief process when you give up something you loved more than anything else in the world. You may have to give up friends who use or even stay away from certain relatives. You may have to end a relationship with a boyfriend or girlfriend who is an active addict. There may be places you historically associated with fun that you must now avoid.

Then there is the loss due to your addictive behaviors prior to recovery. Addicts lose all sorts of important stuff: wife, husband, fiancé, boyfriend, girlfriend, child custody, money, jobs, professional licenses, houses, cars, friends, freedom, etc., etc.

Right about now you are probably wondering if there is any good news. Well, there is. PAWS will resolve with time. Remember that "book study" on the promises I talked about at the beginning of this book? Those promises can come true for you too. You can have real happiness as opposed to that temporary artificial, drug-induced, pseudo-happy feeling that you were constantly seeking but never really finding with drugs. Every minute you are sober, your brain is healing, and you are breaking that horrific hold the drugs had on you. It may be hard to see right now, but serenity and happiness are at the end of that PAWS tunnel.

Recovery is a process not an event. You can learn to address life appropriately and develop trust in your ability to deal with problems without drugs. This will happen only if you are honest during treatment. Honesty will allow you to assess feedback related to your actions and feelings. You must learn to set and keep personal boundaries and respect those of others. You need to unlearn addict behaviors and replace them with healthy, adaptive behaviors like patience, tolerance, mutual respect. If "co-occurring disorders such as depression, anxiety, ADHD, Bipolar Disorders, PTSD, or others are identified, appropriate medications will be prescribed. However, if the addiction is not addressed successfully and put into remission, treatment for any other issue is doomed to failure.

Here are some additional tips to help get through PAWS. Educate yourself so that you will understand what is happening to you. You do not need unrealistic expectations that can result in disappointment based relapse. You do not need to carry around a façade that "everything is fine now." It is also important to stay active and socialize within healthy peer groups. You also need to celebrate your recovery milestones. If craving becomes a major issue, talk about it in a safe environment (no war stories). There are also medications that can help with craving. We have previously discussed many of them and they are available if you need them. There is one anti-craving medication I would like to discuss in a little detail. It is named baclofen.

Baclofen

Baclofen (trade name Lioresal) is classified as a muscle relaxant, but there is growing evidence that it can be beneficial for people seeking recovery from addictive diseases. While the specific mechanism of its action has not been fully determined, it appears to act on GABA-B receptors. What that means is that baclofen dampens the release of dopamine. Dopamine is the main "reward" chemical in our brains. It is the chemical that makes us feel good or "high."

If you have the brain disease of addiction, there is abundant evidence that when you have a craving for a drug, the reward center in your brain gets primed with a small release of internal dopamine. This small release is due to the fact that thinking about the use of your drug of choice is pleasurable. The anticipation of that pleasure is what primes the pump. Baclofen dampens the release of the small amount of dopamine that is the pump primer. You can think of baclofen as a sort of "buzz kill." If baclofen dampens the primer, the craving or urge to use is not as powerful, and relapse is less tempting.

Animal studies indicate that baclofen decreases self-administration of ethanol, nicotine, cocaine, methamphetamine, and heroin.

Clinically, baclofen tends to ease withdrawal symptoms in

both alcohol detox and opiate detox. It is one of the mainstay medications that I prescribe when treating opiate addicts going through detox. There is growing evidence that baclofen can help addicts stay abstinent from opiates once acute detox is complete.

Not only does baclofen help dampen the physiological process of craving, it decreases the opiate high if you do relapse. It also decreases some of the symptoms of PAWS such as anxiety. While it is not an antidepressant, it may still decrease some of the depression commonly seen with PAWS.

Baclofen may also reduce alcohol craving. For that matter, there is clinical evidence that it may reduce cocaine craving.

This is not surprising. We know that all drugs ultimately impact similar brain circuits to give the reward feeling (high). If baclofen is acting on such common addictive circuits, it should not matter what drug activated the circuit. It is the circuit activation that makes the high happen. If we dampen that circuit with baclofen there is less high and less desire to keep on using.

For those of us who do not like neurophysiology, let us look at it another way. Let us say we have five different light switches hooked up to one light, and we will make it so that any switch can turn on the light. The light will serve as the brain. Now, we will label each switch. Switch number one is heroin; switch number two is alcohol; switch number three is cocaine, etc. Most addicts have one switch they like to use more than others, so you can label that switch as your drug of choice.

As noted above we will label the light as "brain," and we will be a little more specific and label it "brain reward."

With this set up, it does not matter if we turn the cocaine switch on or the heroin switch on, as any one of them will push electricity to the light and the light will go on. The reward center lights up brightly.

If we can decrease the amount of electrical power that can get to the light, no matter what switch is turned on, the light will not get as bright. You can flip those switches all you want, but the light is not going to get any brighter. That is how baclofen acts. It decreased the power of the chemical high.

Scientific research on baclofen as an adjunct to the treatment of alcoholism is showing promise. In one particular study, one group of alcoholics took baclofen and one group did not. If you were in the baclofen group, your chance of recovery was seventy percent. If you were in the group that did not take the baclofen, your recovery chance was twenty-four percent. Granted this is only one study, but it points the way for more research into the benefits of this medication.

So what's the down side of baclofen? Well, for one thing, the use of baclofen to treat addictions is an off-label use. That means baclofen is not officially approved for treatment of substance use disorders, but the research indicates it is beneficial.

Another downside is that although it has a low abuse potential (when is the last time you bought baclofen on the street?), it can cause physical dependency. As with anything else, some people will abuse it and get into trouble. This means that abrupt withdrawal of high doses of baclofen can result in seizures and hallucinations.

Side Effects: As with every medication, you must weigh the risks of the undesirable side effects against the benefit of taking the medication. Baclofen can make you drowsy and can cause gastrointestinal problems such as nausea, vomiting, constipation. It can also cause headaches and dizziness. These effects usually go away within a short time.

Baclofen has some other positive "side effects." Baclofen helps with gastroesophageal reflux disease (GERD) and with hiccups.

Dosage: I generally start by prescribing 10 mg of baclofen to be taken three times a day. I will increase the dosage to 20 mg three times per day if needed, but I do that over a five-day period. Some of the research is showing 20 mg three times a day is a good dosage for not only increasing the time a person stays in a treatment program, but also for decreasing the rate of relapse. There are some studies that support higher doses, but that must be very individualized. Monitoring by an addictionologist is a very good idea. This is not a stand-alone treatment for addictions. It is merely a tool that may be applicable in a particular patient and/or situation. It is a biological tool, but no medication is a substitute for the other keys to recovery:
social, psychological, spiritual.

NUTRIENTS AND RECOVERY

Vitamin D is important to all of us and has particular significance in people suffering from addictions. Low levels of Vitamin D can result in a variety of conditions that aggravate mood and pain disorders which increases the risk of relapse and decreases the quality of recovery.

There appears to be an association between low Vitamin D levels and depression. This may be a significant factor in Seasonal Affective Disorder. Low Vitamin D levels also have neurological consequences and may even have implications in dementia. Needless to say, any additional brain damaging factor is absolutely the last thing an addicted brain needs. Trust me when I tell you that we do ample damage with the toxic chemicals we ingested compulsively.

Vitamin D can also impact how we experience pain. A low Vitamin D level can cause pain in muscles, joints, and bones. It also makes pain medications less effective. As a matter of reference, opioid dependent pain patients with low Vitamin D require twice the amount of opiates to control pain as those with normal D levels. Low Vitamin D levels also cause muscle weakness and promote musculoskeletal deconditioning.

How do people get Vitamin D deficiency? Obviously, the level can decrease simply by not taking in enough of it, but there is another risk factor that I am seeing more and more in my addicted patients. That factor is the gastric bypass. It appears that people who have gastric bypass are at more risk for addictions. They are also more at risk for Vitamin D deficiency and consequences like osteoporosis.

I check Vitamin D levels in chronic pain patients and in gastric bypass patients. If the levels are low, replacement with high doses can correct the problem and the symptoms, but the levels must be monitored during replacement therapy because too much Vitamin D can be toxic. Please do not go loading up on Vitamin D because you think you might have a shortage of it.

Folate is a water soluble B vitamin that is an important nutrient for addicts. Low folate is associated with depression and also poor response to antidepressant medications. Folate must be metabolized to L-methylfolate (MTHF) to pass through the blood brain barrier and get into the brain. Some people do not metabolize folate into MTHF as efficiently as others. There are also several medications that interfere with this transition of folate to MTHF. These include Depakote, Lamictal, metformin, and birth control pills. Treatment with MTHF will increase the concentration of MTHF in the brain and can increase response to antidepressant medications.

Omega 3 Fatty Acids are often decreased in patients with ADHD, dementias, and depression. These are essential nutrients that possess anti-inflammatory properties. They can help with pain, brain function, menstrual pain, hypertension, and even decrease cancer risks. However, high doses can also cause you to bleed more easily and increase your risk for hemorrhage.

N-acetylcystine (NAC) is a drug and nutritional supplement. (I know that may sound strange.) It is prescribed for several medical uses such as an antidote for acetaminophen overdose and a medication for breaking up mucous in the lungs and more. The side effect profile is relatively limited, but there are adverse effects, so be informed if you plan on taking it.

NAC may have benefit in some mental diseases including schizophrenia, Bipolar Disorder, Obsessive Compulsive Disorder, anxiety, and depression. It may decrease craving of some addictive drugs and may decrease compulsive gambling behavior. The way it works involves balancing glutamate which is involved in drug craving and withdrawal. Incidentally, glutamate may also be a component of some of the mental illnesses listed above.

We know glutamate balance is a critical component in the withdrawal syndrome due to its properties of "excitotoxicity." Excitotoxicity is one way in which the alcohol and drug withdrawal process itself can cause nerve damage. If a nerve cell gets too over-amped, it can die. This is also one of the reasons cold turkey is a bad choice for detox. We know glutamate excitotoxicity can damage the developing fetus if mom is detoxing from opiates. Indeed, that is one of the reasons we do a very gradual detox process in pregnant addicts.

On the other end of the scale, if we do not have enough glutamate function, our brains are under activated.

Those of us who have experienced craving know we tend to get excited at the prospect of using. That is why we call it a trigger. We get a cue to use, and we get animated and ready for action. Unfortunately, that action may be to get and take the mood-altering substance. We also get that little taste of dopamine from our brain's reward center. If we could dampen that excitation phase, we could decrease the craving. (As previously mentioned, this is probably how baclofen works: to decrease craving.) Please note that I did not say we could stop the craving. Craving has other components besides the glutamate surge, but if you have ever been there in the midst of that overwhelming compulsion, you know that anything that could safely decrease that urge to use is worth a try. I believe NAC can help overcome the compulsion to use.

The usual "dosage" is 1200 mg twice a day. I see no benefit in going over that amount. Indeed, there is some indication that too much NAC may have the opposite effect. If you are still into thinking like an addict, "If one is good, ten or more must be better," you are wrong! Stick with the 1200 mg twice a day and talk about it with your addictionologist or primary care doctor before you start it.

Vitamins: My patients frequently ask me to suggest a good vitamin for them. I usually recommend a basic multivitamin but with some precautions. The latest research is showing that too much calcium might actually promote hardening and narrowing of arteries so I stay on the low end of taking any extra calcium supplements. There is also concern that taking extra (supplemental) Vitamin E and/or selenium (a trace element) actually increases the risk for the development of prostate cancer.

A healthy diet will cover most vitamin requirements. I will admit that I do take a little extra Vitamin C especially during the flu season.

Choline: Let me start off by saying I take choline daily. True to form, there is a story as to how I arrived at my decision to take choline. Here it is. The National Academy of Science declares choline as essential for normal cell function. Nutritionally, choline is grouped in with the B vitamins. It directly affects nerve cells and is needed for normal nerve cell signaling.

During pregnancy, choline is essential for normal brain development and memory function. As a matter of fact it is essential for the development of the hippocampus which we have talked about earlier. Since COAs and survivors of severe stress seem to have a possibility for hippocampal damage, supplementation with choline seems reasonable.
Choline can improve memory function even in healthy adult brains. Many addictive drugs impair memory function, and while memory function tends to improve with time and abstinence, choline may speed up the process. There is also

research to support some protective effects on memory in the aging brain.

So, given the facts that I am a recovering addict and I am an ACOA and I am not getting any younger, I take choline. There are other pertinent facts that support making sure you have enough choline if you are in recovery.

Adequate choline intake helps treat some forms of liver disease including Hepatitis C. By decreasing "oxidative stress," choline may help limit the development of scar tissue in the liver and by definition decrease the development of liver cirrhosis.

Choline may also enhance nerve transmission to muscle tissue.
Choline may also help decrease anxiety.

Choline has anti-inflammatory properties. It can decrease inflammation in the lungs of people who suffer from asthma and can decrease the number and severity of asthma attacks.

Having said all that, choline is not a miracle nutrient. You are not going to develop a photographic memory over night because you took some choline. Memory improvements may be subtle. The idea is to protect your brain from additional loss or at least greatly slow the process down. Men require more choline that women.

A supplemental dose of 500 to 1000 mg per day seems reasonable especially since a "normal" diet probably contains an adequate amount of choline. I take 500 mg a day.

Too much choline can have undesirable side effects. One of them is that you start to smell like fish which is not exactly an endearing quality unless you happen to be "the crazy cat lady" of the neighborhood and are trying to attract felines.

To make it even worse, you sweat a lot, salivate or slobber a lot, and vomit a lot. High doses can also cause blood pressure to drop. If you decide to take choline supplements, let your doctor know about it.

Chocolate: If you have been in my office at the detox center, you know I try to keep a bowl of chocolate candy available for "visitors." Dark chocolate, in moderation, really is good for you and for me! It may help those screaming opiate receptors during opiate detox. Cocoa may help brain function by increasing blood flow to the brain especially if you are older, like me. Looks like I qualify for dark chocolate and a couple of cups of hot chocolate a day. ☺

"USP" REFERS TO U.S. PHARMACOPEIAL CONVENTION WHICH IS A NONPROFIT ORGANIZATION THAT SETS STANDARDS FOR THE PURITY OF DIETARY SUPPLEMENTS. I ADVISE YOU TO ALWAYS MAKE SURE USP APPROVAL IS DOCUMENTED ON ANY SUPPLEMENT YOU TAKE.

FUTURE OF ADDICTION TREATMENT MEDICATION

Researchers are actively looking for ways to treat addictions. Addiction a big problem and it is also big business for the pharmaceutical companies. So, buyer beware!

Here are some of the things going on currently:

Nalmefene (Revex): This drug is similar to naltrexone. It's nothing new. It was initially used for the treatment of opiate overdose. It came out in the1970's for addictions treatment and sort of just went away. The brand name is no longer available in the USA. There is some work going on to make a long-lasting injectable form. It may have some advantages over naltrexone. The big question is not just when it will get to the USA market, but if it will get to the market. Between the FDA processes and competing pharmaceutical companies, you never really know what will happen.

THC Patch or the "marijuana patch": There is a drug company working on a THC skin patch. The plan, as I understand it, is to use it to treat marijuana detox and/or marijuana dependency. I am not a big fan of maintenance "therapy" for addiction treatment. The patch is also expected to be useful in cancer patients and HIV-infected patients. It is not available yet.

Kudzu Treatment: Yep! Kudzu! We all know about kudzu. It is the plant that grows all over everything. Kudzu use goes back about 1400 or so years when it was used by the Chinese as a hangover remedy. A rather limited study at Harvard indicated that Kudzu extract appears to reduce the amount of alcohol ingested during a drinking session. The active ingredient is evidently puerarin. It did not stop drinking, but in this study it did reduce it modestly. There is some concern that the way it decreased the amount of alcohol consumed was by increasing the rate alcohol got into the brain. In other words, you might get drunker, faster so you would drink a little less. At any rate, I would not jump out of my car and start gnawing on kudzu leaves at this point, but I will watch the research and get back to you.

New Targets: More and more research into addictions will lead to medications that specifically target various brain chemicals and nerve receptors. Some may target specific sites on your chromosomes to prevent misreading of your DNA. but nothing works better than "not picking up" the drug in the first place.

About Those Drug Companies

Pharmaceutical companies exist to make money. I have no problem with that. What I have a problem with is the fact that some pharmaceutical companies unethically, immorally, and illegally promote addictive substances which in turn promote addiction. Many people have the idea that if a medication is approved by government and prescribed by doctors, it must be okay to take. That seems reasonable especially in the United States of America. Sadly, that is not always the case. Subsequently, I feel the need to shine the light on some pharmaceutical company activities that clearly violate that intent and trust.

Let us start with the Purdue Pharma Company, makers of OxyContin. Unless you are a hermit living in a cave somewhere, you know about OxyContin and how additive it is. However, you may not know how it became so readily available and got so popular.

The name origin of OxyContin is interesting. The "Oxy" part refers to the drug itself which is pure oxycodone. The "Contin" part refers to the properties of the oxycodone formulation which makes the drug's effect continuous or long acting nature.

OxyContin addiction became established due to a criminal behavior perpetrated Purdue Pharma called "misbranding." Purdue promoted the drug to doctors as having a lower abuse potential than other opioids such as Percodan and Lortab. The lower addiction potential was based on its time-release formulation.

When I say "promoted", I mean they launched an aggressive marketing campaign, and they targeted doctors with little experience in true pain management and with apparently even less experience in the risks of addiction. Purdue's immoral, unethical, and illegal marketing ploys worked.

OxyContin was responsible for ninety percent of Purdue's revenue. Just to give you an idea of how corrupt this mislabeling campaign was, I want to give you just one example. Purdue let their marketers draw fake scientific charts to give to doctors. These fake charts "showed" how OxyContin had a low abuse potential. Seriously!

Pain patients were subsequently prescribed the medication by misled doctors who purportedly thought the drug was less addictive than other opiates. They were wrong. Addiction to "Oxy" became commonplace. The drug soon became "popular" on the street. Addicts would crush it up and snort it nasally or inject it intravenously. By doing this, they bypassed the long acting formulation and got an immediate rush of euphoria which was relatively short acting. More than one of my patients refer to as "legal heroin."

While it took addicts no time at all to realize how addictive Oxy was, it took the government six years to figure it all out and to hold Purdue responsible for its crimes. Six years is a long time, and that accounted for lots of new addicts (including teenagers) and dead addicts and destroyed lives and damaged families before the government finally stepped in.

In federal court, Purdue Pharma company executives admitted to fraudulently promoting the drug for six years as being less prone to abuse and having fewer narcotic side effects than other opioids. In short, they intentionally lied.

Purdue ended up paying a fine of over six hundred million dollars. Three top executives including the president, the top company lawyer, and the medical director paid fines and pled guilty to criminal charges. They got off with doing community service instead of jail time.

Purdue reformulated the OxyContin so that it cannot be crushed or dissolved without turning into a gummy type substance, but my patients tell me there are ways to get around this.

There is more bad news. Since then, the FDA has approved another long-acting opiate, Zohydro, which is pure hydrocodone. The FDA went against the recommendations of its expert advisory panel that wanted the FDA to reject the drug. The expert advisory panel voted eleven to two against approval of this opioid. Amazingly, the FDA overrode that opinion. This new "disaster in the making" has sent its company's stock soaring, and attorneys generals from 28 states are asking the FDA to reconsider the drug's approval.

By the way, it is not just the drug companies and the FDA we need to worry about betraying us. The Walgreens drugstore chain was recently fined eighty-eight million dollars by the Drug Enforcement Administration (DEA) because it allowed millions of controlled drugs, including oxycodone, to reach illegal markets. Two Walgreens drugstores in Florida reportedly each pushed 2.2 million pills out the doors each year. That is a lot of dope dealing!

SLEEP AND SUBSTANCE USE DISORDERS

There are numerous reasons why some, if not most, addicts (recovering and otherwise) have sleep problems. The most obvious reason is the chemical disruption and imbalance in the brain caused by the intake of mood-altering chemicals in an excessive and compulsive manner. Even after acute detoxification from an addictive substance, sleep issues persist and may do so for months. As previously stated, it takes months, if not years, for the brain to heal and "recalibrate." On top of that, many "recovering addicts" continue their addiction to cigarettes. Notice that I said cigarettes and not just nicotine. (See cigarette/nicotine section for clarity.) Many addicts have sleep apnea. Then there is GERD (Gastro-Esophageal Reflux Disease) which can make a night miserable. Some addicts have nightmares and using dreams. Some addicts suffer from Post-Traumatic Stress Disorders (PTSD) and bedtime is "fear time."

Restless Leg Syndrome (RLS) is a frequent complaint in my patient population. This is a neurological condition involving the neurotransmitter dopamine. Dopamine is the main neurotransmitter involved in opiate dependency and in withdrawal. RLS can be a separate syndrome that presents clinically as the need to move the legs especially at night when trying to sleep. There are effective medications for RLS. Ropinirole (trade name Requip) is pretty effective. Some people respond to pramipexole (Mirapex). Gabapentin (Neurontin) is a good option that also helps with anxiety and with alcohol or benzodiazepine detox, and clonidine (Catapres) has the added benefit of decreasing opiate withdrawal symptoms. Smoking cigarettes is associated with RLS as well as generalized sleep problems.

In the "old days" as in 1978 when I entered treatment, the solution to sleeplessness was to memorize the Big Book.

While that seemed like sound advice at the time, we now know the correction of sleep rhythms is important for generalized wellbeing. Besides that, insomnia is often a relapse trigger.

Addicts typically complain of two major sleep issues. One is *"I cannot get to sleep."* This is called prolonged sleep latency. The other common problem is *"I wake up all during the night."* This is called fragmented sleep. You can have both prolonged latency and fragmented sleep.

Medications: There are certain non-addictive medications that are useful in helping normalize sleep patterns. These are considered "mood stabilizers." These medications are NOT mood-altering. Use of mood-altering chemicals is how we got addicted in the first place. The idea behind these medications is not brain alteration but brain stabilization and recovery.

Use of mood stabilizers helps you heal. As your brain heals, you and your doctor may decide to begin tapering medications. This is something to discuss with your health care provider. I advise against stopping medications on your own. We both know where being your own prescriber got you.

There are two points to consider about sleep medication: (1) restorative sleep is the goal and (2) passing out is not sleep.

With all this in mind, let us have a look at some medication options.

We will start with **Seroquel (quetiapine)**. This used to be a rather expensive drug but the quick acting form has recently "gone generic" and is more affordable. It is classified as an atypical antipsychotic that has sedative effects. Seroquel is used to treat schizophrenia, bipolar disorder, and major depression. Interestingly, Seroquel may have a positive effect on addiction treatment outcomes. No one is really sure why it does this. It could improve outcomes simply because it improves sleep and has some antidepressant effects. Research continues.

If you have "racing thoughts" this might be the one for you. I start at a low dose and titrate upward as needed. I start with 25 mg or 50 mg at night, and I rarely prescribe over 200 mg per night. Now as I say that, if a person has Bipolar Disorder, the evening Seroquel dose may be higher. The maximal beneficial dose in such instances is generally considered 400 mg but some healthcare providers go higher.

As with any medication there are pros and cons. Weight gain is a big "con" for many people. Seroquel can even lead to a condition called metabolic syndrome which consists of excess body fat, high blood sugar (diabetes), and high blood pressure. Not everyone gains weight on Seroquel, but some people do. There is a way to combat the weight gain and that is by prescribing metformin which is actually a medication for diabetes.

Some people complain of a hangover feeling from Seroquel. If that is the case, we can either lower the dosage or stop the medication. I prescribe it on an as needed (PRN) basis. Most people wean off of it within a few weeks or so. I have never seen a Seroquel, addict but there are reports of Seroquel abuse in prison environments.

Trazadone is an antidepressant that has strong sedation properties at low doses. Indeed, the main side effect of trazadone is drowsiness, so that works out well. You might also experience dry mouth and dizziness initially. The usual starting dose is 50 mg at night. The dosage can be increased up to 200 mg at night if needed. I have never had to go to 200 mg. Trazadone helps you go to sleep and thereby shortens the latency part of the problem. It also decreases the tendency to awaken during the night and thereby helps with sleep fragmentation. Trazodone tends to provide restorative sleep which improves your overall mood and thinking capability. In my experience, patients rarely complain of any hangover effect. Of course, trazodone is not for everyone. Some people tell me it gives them vivid and disturbing dreams. However there is one particular side effect in males that is very uncommon in my experience of prescribing this drug, but since even uncommon side effects occur, we need to talk about it. That side effect is priapism.

Priapism is a condition in which the penis becomes engorged with blood and this causes an erection which can be painful. The standard definition includes a time line of having a sustained erection for over four hours, but this seems rather arbitrary to me. Priapism is a medical emergency and treatment can range from icepacks and/or medications to actual surgical procedures. In the two cases I have witnessed, stopping the trazodone resolved the problem. I suspect one of the reasons I do not see the side effect of priapism as often as it is predicted in the literature (one out of every six thousand patents) is because of the low doses I prescribe.

> *There is a case report in one of the psychiatry journals about a male patient who went to the hospital due to priapism and had it successfully treated with a minor shunt procedure on his penis. However, he evidently did not bother to tell the hospital doctors that he was on trazodone at the time. He also did not show up for his medical follow up appointment. He did however resume taking the trazodone. As a matter of fact, he reportedly doubled the dose to 300 mg at night. He evidently had a clotting disease also. Long story short, he had another severe case of priapism, and his penis had to be amputated. I mention this rare case only because*

it is a rather succinct example as to why a patient should not increase the dosage of this medication on his own accord, or take someone else's medication, or give someone else his medication, or not be forthcoming with any healthcare provider who is treating him, or not keep follow up appointments. If you want to read the story yourself, check it out at The Primary Care Companion to the Journal of Clinical Psychiatry 2010 12(2) under Penile Amputation After Trazodone-Induced Priapism: A Case Report.

Combination of Seroquel and Trazodone: Use of low doses of both of these drugs in combination is an option if taking just one of them does not work well.

Amitriptyline (Elavil) is a sedating tricyclic antidepressant (TCA). I think it is only available as a generic now. It has been around so long that the patent is probably gone away, but the trade name, Elavil, has stuck around. I tend to stay away from Elavil during acute detoxification simply because it can increase the risk of seizures during alcohol or benzodiazepine withdrawal. Elavil has many uses other than treatment of depression. It may help with the treatment of chronic pain. It, too, causes dry mouth and may make it difficult to urinate. As always, if I prescribe it, I start at a relatively low dose (10 to 25 mg at night). It is not a good choice in older alcoholics for a variety of reasons such as fall risk and problems with thinking straight.

Doxepin is another TCA that at doses of 1 to 6 mg taken 30 minutes prior to sleep and on an empty stomach can promote getting to sleep, and there is no hangover the next day and is not associated with weight gain.

Mirtazapine (Remeron) is an antidepressant that helps some recovering addicts sleep. I start with 15 mg at night and will increase it up to 30 mg at night. Again, the major side effect is drowsiness, which is why it is used as a sleep agent. Of course there are other side effects including the possibility of increased appetite and weight gain.

Hydroxyzine (Vistaril) came out in the 1950's as an antihistamine. It is pretty good for nausea too. As it turns out, lower doses are good for anxiety treatment and higher doses can put you to sleep. Plus, it is not addicting. It does not work for everyone but then again what does?

Melatonin is a "neurohormone" produced by your pineal gland which is located in the middle of your brain and looks sort of like a little pine cone. Your pineal gland is like a little internal clock. Melatonin can decrease the time it takes you to get to sleep (sleep latency). It may also help you get back into some semblance of a normal circadian sleep rhythm. Dosage is between 1 to 5 mg about an hour before bedtime.

I had one patient who was very concerned that I was offering him a medication that would "mess with" his pineal gland. He had some not-so-scientific perceptions about the pineal. There seems to be a large body of information on the subject which one might find interesting. Let us take a very brief look at some of the pineal lore.

This little pea-sized gland has been the source of some long-standing and fascinating controversy. Ancient Egyptians attributed spiritual and psychic powers to it. They may have considered it to be "The Eye of the god Horus." Descartes, the Father of Philosophy, declared in the 1600's that the pineal gland was the "seat of the soul." Wow! Others believed it to be the "Third Eye" which was our gateway into the spiritual plane. With a finely tuned pineal gland, you could astral project into other dimensions. Needless to say, this line of thought can be popular with a certain type of hallucinogen addict.

There is also a school of thought that the world governments are pumping fluoride into the water, not to help you build strong teeth, but to kill the pineal's third eye capability. I am not convinced by any of this, but I love reading it, and I ask the reader's pardon for this little digression. I do agree that the pineal gland is important in regulating our sleep cycles and that we have medications that target that effect.

Let us proceed.

Ramelteon (Rozerem) is a melatonin mimic that can help you fall asleep. I do not prescribe it much since it may increase a hormone called prolactin and it can decrease testosterone. Prolactin is the hormone that impacts sexual function. Many people I treat are addicted to opiates. Opiates decrease the testosterone levels and increase prolactin levels. I do not want to make that worse.

Passion Flower Tea comes from the Passiflora incarnate plant. This really is the only "herbal" preparation that I credit with having a decent scientific basis for helping with sleep. I recommend it and I have it on hand for my acute detox patients and my post-acute detox patients. At the risk of another digression, I do want to note that the name "Passion Flower" refers to the Passion of Christ, and the flower symbolizes that Passion. It is not an aphrodisiac. It was named by 17th century Spanish priests who were in South America at the time. There is one final caveat. A cup of Passion Flower tea is the proper dosage. There is no need to glug down a gallon. Stick with one cup at night.

Sleep hygiene is important. Obviously, addicts are used to grabbing a drug to cure all ills. While the above medications can help, it is not a good idea to rely on them as the only way to sleep. Sleep hygiene includes establishing a sleep schedule, having a pre-sleep ritual (like a warm bath), avoiding caffeine for six hours or so prior to sleep time, avoiding the stimulant nicotine, not exercising right before going to bed, not binging on food, doing some relaxation techniques, having a peaceful sleep environment and a comfortable bed.

Night Sweats are common in the early days of detoxification especially from opiates, but night sweats can also persist after detox. The cause in those cases may remain undetermined. Several things can cause the problem including acute anxiety, chronic anxiety, and/or depression. Some antidepressants can actually cause night sweats. Most night sweating is worse in the early morning hours. A trial course of Catapres is worth a try, and some of my patients report a good response to this medication. Catapres is a pretty good choice if the night sweats are part of a Post-Acute Withdrawal Process.

Post-Traumatic Stress Disorder and Nightmares: The use of prazosin in doses starting from 1 mg and going up to 4 mg can give relief from PTSD nightmares. Prazosin (trade name Minipress) is a medication used to treat high blood pressure, but it has proven to be beneficial in PTSD nightmares. I recommend starting at 1 mg at night and giving it a few nights to work. If needed, increase it by an additional 1 mg for a few more nights and reassess again. In my clinical experience, there has not been the need to increase the dose above 3 mg at night. I have noted pretty good clinical results with this approach.

CO-OCCURRING DISORDERS

Anxiety and Substance Use Disorder

A co-occurring disorder is just that. You have one diagnosis, which is addiction in our case, and you also have some other additional diagnosis such as anxiety, depression, ADHD, and/or Bipolar Disorder to name a few.

Anxiety is a major co-occurring disorder in many addicts. Untreated anxiety can also be a major relapse trigger. The diagnosis cannot be accurately made during detox or in the very early days of recovery since every addict in detox is anxious. Then there is the anxiety that often accompanies a post-acute withdrawal syndrome (PAWS). This type of anxiety can last for months, but it eases up over time (that would be sober time). I inform addicts that in early recovery it is not unexpected to experience some anxiety from PAWS as well as from living in the real world without drugs. We offer some specific CBT skills to address PAWS anxiety, and if needed, we can prescribe appropriate medications for such anxiety.

Research continues to clarify the links between anxiety, addiction, and relapse. We are going to delve a little into brain function and physiology, and with the help of the latest research, try to explain some of these connections. Clearly, I think an understanding of this is important to addicts as well as anyone who is prescribed medications such as benzodiazepines for anxiety.

Chronic use of alcohol has a long-lasting impact on the user's level of stress and ability to handle stress. Alcohol and/or other sedative/hypnotic drugs (such as benzodiazepines, SOMA, etc.) actually cause the brain to shift its stress response mechanisms. Frequent use of alcohol causes frequent recalibrations of those stress survival mechanisms. This recalibration process causes "wear and tear" on the brain which ultimately results in an abnormal stress response. I will not get too deeply into all the nuances, but this alcohol/drug-induced stress impacts the brain's "central stress response network."

That central network is called the HPA (Hypothalamic-Pituitary-Adrenal) axis. We can see from the name that the brain stress system has a connection between the brain and the adrenal glands. The adrenals sit on top of each kidney. Indeed the name ad-renal means to add something (in this case a gland) to the kidney. These little glands secrete stress hormones that help initiate a "fight or flight or freeze" response to a real or imagined threat. Here is how it works:

We will say you are walking down the street, and suddenly a huge angry, bare-fanged dog that is frothing at the mouth charges you. Your HPA axis is immediately activated. It, in turn, activates your adrenal glands. You immediately run away (**flight**) from the mad animal, or you pick up a weapon and **fight** the creature, or you **freeze** in fear. This happens in seconds. You do not think about it. You react! This is a good thing. If a rabid dog charges you, this is not be the time to start thinking. "Hmmm. I see an angry dog charging me. Hmmm. He is frothing at the mouth. Hmmm. That could be rabies. Hmmm. He might bite me." By that time it would all be over, and you would be in an ambulance or in the morgue.

Now, once this HPA axis goes on full alert, it also calms down back to normal when the stress is over. That way, you are ready just in case another threat comes along. It is a great system, but it is also one we can mess up with alcohol or other drugs. (Other things such as child abuse, major trauma, etc., can disrupt it also.)

Can you imagine always being on full alert and fearful? It

would be like constantly waiting for that mad dog to come at you any moment. Can you imagine little stressors setting you off and causing a racing heart, shortness of breath, and the need to run away? Can you imagine being so afraid of normal things that you dread them or avoid then altogether?

If you have a disrupted and stressed out HPA axis, not only can you imagine it, you live it.

If you use alcohol or certain other drugs on a chronic basis, you can definitely stress your HPA axis out. What the person with these changes experiences is a negative emotional state with symptoms such as such as increased anxiety, changes in sleep, changes in appetite, aggressive behaviors, agitated behaviors, changes in concentration, changes in memory, and most germane to our conversation, increased desire for the use of alcohol or other mood-altering drugs (relapse).

> *"I am always afraid I will have an anxiety attack. I cannot sleep because I just lay there and worry all night. I cannot seem to turn it off unless I drink or take a Xanax. That works a little while then it comes back. Little things set me off. It is almost as if I look for things to worry about."* Lenny, 32-year-old with diagnosis of Substance use Disorder and Generalized Anxiety Disorder.

Lenny is caught in a trap. He is not drinking or taking Xanax to feel good. He is taking it to ward off negative feelings. (We call this negative reinforcement.)However, the booze and/or Xanax only give him temporary relief, and as he escalates the doses, he makes things worse for this HPA axis.

The end result from this recurrent chemical storm is that a certain stress hormone (Cortisol) in your brain shifts to account for the drug effect. You end up being more sensitive to stress and if you do happened to active your HPA axis, it takes longer for the Cortisol to get back to a normal base. In other words you stay in a state of anxiety longer than the person who does not use alcohol or drugs. You are what my grandmother used to call a "nervous person" or a "worry wart."

Interestingly, too much or too little Cortisol impairs your ability to formulate memories. That means you are more prone to maintain habits (such as drinking) rather than learn new goal-directed processes. Here is another interesting observation. Naltexone (Vivitrol and others) tends to help normalize the Cortisol levels in alcoholics and addicts during early recovery. This may be one of the reasons it helps decrease cravings. One more pearl is that research has shown that an abnormal cortisol response is a predictor that the person will relapse.

The HPA axis in interconnected with a plethora of other brain structures though a plethora of networks. Therefore, you will not be surprised to learn that other systems get out of whack. For instance, the blue spot in your brain (locus coeruleus) can secrete too much norepinephrine and cause or worsen your state of anxiety. If one of the reasons for your anxiety is that your "blue spot" is out of whack, a medication that was developed to treat high blood pressure (clonidine) can help decrease your anxiety. It does this by calming the "blue spot" down so you don't over-amp on the norepinephrine.

There is another "antihypertensive" drug by the name of prazosin (trade name Minipress) that reduces the stress response and may decrease alcohol relapse. As you will recall, it is also good for treating nightmares.

Lots of other brain chemicals get disrupted (dopamine, NPY, serotonin, endocannabinoids), but that is beyond the scope of this discussion.

So why is it important that we talk about all this? Well, first of all, you need to be informed about what is going on in your brain and the rest of your body when you use alcohol and/or other drugs. And secondly, you need to know what to expect early on in recovery, so you are better prepared to deal with PAWS. You also need to know why we make certain treatment/recovery recommendations to you.

1. After acute detox, your stress response system is going to be raw for about 12 weeks. It will continue to heal (if you let it), but the first 12 weeks seem to be the worst.
2. Detox plus 12 weeks adds up to right at 90 days. This is a high-risk time for relapse. This is also another clinical rationale for an initial 90-day treatment experience.
3. Your reward system is also going to be out of tilt for months.
4. If you do use alcohol and/or other drugs during this time, not only do you stop the healing process, you go back to ground zero or possibly even worse.
5. You need to employ recovery tools to deal with this anxiety. Specific medications may help you heal.
6. Cigarette smoking has an adverse impact on the HPA axis. This may be part of the reason cigarette smokers are more prone to relapse than non-smokers.

Primary Anxiety Disorders: Even in the face of substance-induced anxiety, a diagnosis of an independent anxiety disorder can be determined. There are clinical clues that raise the index of probability for a diagnosis of an anxiety disorder. If the onset of anxiety occurred prior to involvement with mood-altering chemicals and/or the symptoms of anxiety disorder occur during periods of significant sobriety or abstinence, the clinician must suspect an independent anxiety disorder diagnosis. It is also important to inquire about a family history of anxiety or any other mood disorder. When doing so, the clinician should ascertain what medications helped those family members with a positive history because the same medications might be helpful to this patient.

Anxiety is not just one disorder. In addition to Generalized Anxiety, there are Social Anxiety, Panic Disorders, Post Traumatic Stress Disorders, and Obsessive Disorders. While treatments of these different types of anxiety disorders share some commonalities, treatments are not the same for all types of anxiety.

The first line of medical therapy for Generalized Anxiety Disorder (GAD) is an elective Serotonin Reuptake Inhibitor antidepressant (**SSRI**). Patients often ask me why I am prescribing an antidepressant for anxiety. While an SSRI is an antidepressant, it also works for anxiety because the brain chemical serotonin can get out of whack if you have an abnormal stress response going on. In short, these medications help correct brain chemical imbalances associated not only with depression but also with anxiety.

There are many SSRI's. They all have some differences and they generally take four to six weeks for the therapeutic effect to really kick in. If you have GAD, it may also take a while to find the one that works best for you. Some anxiety patients may have a positive response to a Serotonin Norepinephrine Reuptake Inhibitor (**SNRI**). There are lots of these medications around, and each one is a little different. Treatment of GAD requires commitment and an ongoing therapeutic relationship with your healthcare provider. Genetic testing may help with the selection of an anti-anxiety medication.

Pregabalin (Lyrica) may have a place in the treatment of GAD. This medication may be worth a try if you've historically taken lots of benzodiazepines (Xanax, Klonopin, etc.). I only say this because some studies have shown pregabalin to be almost as effective as benzodiazepines for anxiety except it does not have the addictive abuse potential of a benzodiazepine. Morever, if you are an addict, you know where the benzos are going to lead you. While Lyrica does not have the addictive abuse potential of the benzodiazepines, there is an abuse potential. It is relatively low, but caution must be exercised to avoid dependency.

Buspiron (Buspar) is another non-addictive anti-anxiety medication. Most addicts with anxiety who have a positive response to this medication do so with higher doses. Buspiron does not work overnight and may take weeks before you see a beneficial result. It does not seem to be of much benefit in Social Anxiety Disorder (SAD) or panic disorder.

Hydroxyzine (Vistaril) can be helpful in decreasing anxiety. I prescribe this on a regular basis for anxiety because it works and it's not addictive. At the same time, I do not want anyone going to Vistaril or any other drug without first trying non-drug techniques to deal with their anxiety.

Propranolol (Inderal) is a beta blocker. What is a beta blocker? Think of it as a drug that blocks that surge of adrenalin you get when you're threatened with harm. By the way, the threat can be real or imagined, but to the person panicking, it is very real. For instance, public speaking is perceived by some people as a threatening experience. Let us say, for example, you do not like to speak in public, but you are in a situation that you cannot get out of and you must do it. You may start to panic, your heart rate goes up, your blood pressure goes up, your muscles start trembling, you have "butterflies" in your stomach, your hands are sweaty, and you are prepared for "flight." Propranolol blocks some of those symptoms and helps you control panicky feelings.

Social anxiety is not uncommon, and you might be surprised at how many people take propranolol before going on stage or doing other scary stuff like meeting their prospective in-laws.

Social Anxiety can also be helped with some of the antidepressant medications and gabapentin.

Clonidine (Catapres) as you know by now is actually a medication for high blood pressure treatment that also offers relief in acute opiate withdrawal. I have found it to be useful in treating anxiety associated with PAWS. It also helps with opiate withdrawal anxiety and with night sweats. I do not prescribe it for anxiety disorders per se unless I think the anxiety is related to PAWS.

Talk Therapy - Cognitive Behavioral Therapy (CBT) aims at addressing harmful thought patterns and ideas related to one's emotions. There are various types but the point here is that CBT helps people deal with anxiety. Medications alone are not the answer, at least in my opinion. In addition to CBT, relaxation techniques and meditation really help control anxiety.

Obsessive Compulsive Thinking: An obsessive thought is one that preoccupies the mind. In the case of a disorder, the thought is usually an unwelcome and unreasonable one that induces fear. A compulsion is a repetitive behavior. If the compulsive behavior is not performed, anxiety is induced. These behaviors include compulsive hand washing, compulsive cleaning, compulsive checking, compulsive counting, and even hoarding. Other compulsive behaviors include hair pulling or trichotillomania, skin picking or dermatillomania, and nail biting or onychophagia. The first line of treatment consists of Cognitive Behavioral Therapy. Medications prescribed to help treat obsessive compulsive behaviors include antidepressants, anticonvulsants, and even antipsychotics.

Interestingly, for some people suffering with OCD, opiates may provide relief of their symptoms. This is turn promotes them to become opiate dependent, like Sharon.

> *"I have been plagued by OCD for years. It makes me miserable, and I get to where I cannot even function. I tried seeing a psychiatrist and a psychologist, but I never could get over it. Then, when I twisted my ankle a few years ago, the doctor gave me some Lortab. When I took it, the obsessive thoughts went away. It was like a miracle. I had to fake pain for a long time to get the hydrocodone, but when that stopped working, I found people to buy it from. I know I'm addicted, but I don't know if I can make it without hydrocodone."*

Thus, OCD appears to be another risk factor for becoming opioid dependent in some individuals.

Attention deficit Disorder and Substance Use Disorder

From my experiences over the years I have come to the conclusion that Attention Deficit Hyperactivity Disorder (ADHD) and Attention Deficit Disorder (ADD) may be just about as misunderstood as Substance Use Disorders (SUDs). There is certainly a growing amount of controversy about the diagnosis and subsequent treatment with addictive stimulant medications. From a symptom and treatment standpoint, I view the ADHD continuum as almost three separate diseases based upon the age group: childhood ADHD, adolescent ADHD, and adult ADHD. Each grouping or phase has unique brain development components, symptoms, and treatment issues. How childhood ADHD is treated (or not treated) will impact adolescent ADHD which in turn will impact adult ADHD.

The basic brain chemical abnormalities of ADHD relate to dopamine, norepinephrine, and glutamate. These are the same brain chemicals that are involved in addiction and addiction treatment.

Unfortunately, some of the medications used to treat ADHD are medications with a high abuse potential, especially amphetamine and amphetamine-like medications. There are self-proclaimed professionals of all sorts who "make a diagnosis" of ADHD using some short checklist. I contend that a checklist is only a screening tool and that a "positive" result indicates a need for legitimate ADHD testing, not for a prescription of a Schedule II addictive substance. The clinical utility of a screen is not for making a diagnosis, it is to indicate who needs additional diagnostic testing. Getting a legitimate diagnosis can really be a convoluted process. Misdiagnosis or over diagnosis often results in being medicated with a dangerous and addictive drug. This is bad not only for the identified patient/victim, but also for those with a legitimate diagnosis.

Whether it be from ignorance, arrogance, impairment, greed, or some other reason, the cavalier prescribing of Adderall has become a major problem.

Before prescribing a controlled, addictive substance to a patient and putting a diagnostic label on that person, it is just good medical practice to have a proper diagnosis. As such, an appropriate assessment by a qualified specialist, inclusive of childhood history, and appropriate diagnostic testing is what I consider to be the standard of care.

Be that as it may, it is relatively easy to get an amphetamine prescription, and there is a whole subculture of college students who are paving their way to addiction via non-medical Adderall. Here is a reality check! Just about anyone can study better with a load of amphetamines on board. It is called "academic doping." What part of "doping" do they not understand?

Over six percent of full-time college students have used Adderall non-medically. Right at eighty percent of those same students used marijuana as compared to thirty percent of non-Adderall users. Almost thirty percent of them used cocaine, and forty-five percent of them used opiates.

If a stimulant medication is indicated, appropriate precaution and monitoring must be in place. A substance use history and a family history must be obtained. A family history of substance use disorders could place the patient at risk if addictive stimulants are prescribed. I wish it was unnecessary to say this, but experience dictates the need to do so, if the patient has a substance use disorder history, I would counsel against prescribing an amphetamine or amphetamine-like stimulant. "First do no harm" is sound advice.

ADHD is more prevalent in SUD patients than in the general population. We do not have the space or time to deal with the reasons in this section. Suffice to say, ADHD is more common in the patient population I treat, and ADHD cannot be ignored. Untreated ADHD lessens the chance for SUD recovery. That does not equate to handing out amphetamines in a treatment center. There are non-addictive medications that can help, but medications alone are not the answer. We need to provide the psycho-social tools to the addict with ADHD to help him or her compensate for the ADHD.

The medications we prescribe most for those who have a co-existing diagnoses of ADHD/ADD and addiction are Strattera and Intuniv.

Atomoxetine (Strattera) causes the brain chemicals norepinephrine and dopamine to be more available and therefore more active. It generally takes Strattera a week or so to kick in. If there is not response after six to eight weeks, it should be discontinued. It only needs to be taken once a day. I usually start with 40 mg per day and can titrate up to 80 mg per day. There is some indication that Strattera may also help control binge eating.

Side Effects: With Strattera, there is an increased risk of suicidal thinking in children and adolescents. There is also the possibility of liver damage. The main things I usually see are dry mouth and even initial drowsiness. However, there are a plethora of side effects to watch for. One side effect which may be beneficial in some patients is that it may help with depression. It does this by improving norepinephrine levels. An attractive effect of atomoxetine in my patient population is that it may decrease impulsive, risk-taking behaviors.

Guanfacine (Intuniv): Is another non-addictive, non-stimulant medication for the treatment of ADHD. It is an alpha2A-adrenergic receptor agonist. You do not need to memorize this, but these types of medications are useful in treating addictions. Intuniv belongs to a "family" of drugs used to treat high blood pressure. It acts on areas of the brain that promote "working memory" and decrease distractibility.

Side Effects: As expected, since this medication is an antihypertensive, some of the side effects include low blood pressure and low heart rate. Drowsiness and light headedness may also occur.

Pros and Cons and Comments: Since Strattera and Intuniv have different mechanisms to treat the same symptoms, a combination of the two might be considered if there is not an adequate response to either one alone. This would be an individualized decision between patient and prescriber and would require dosage adjustments and monitoring.

Bupropion (Wellbutrin) is an antidepressant that has proved to be effective for ADHD in some individuals. The sustained release formulation would be preferred in this situation. This would be an off label use of this medication. An attractive side effect in my patient population is that bupropion may help decrease cigarette smoking.

Omega-3-fatty acid supplements are safe if taken properly and may help as an addition to Strattera and/or Intuniv. Interestingly, a deficiency of omega-3-fatty acids may be seen in various psychiatric disorders including ADHD.

Depression and Substance Use Disorder

Addiction is a downward spiral that can end in oblivion. Along the way we addicts can do a lot of damage. Indeed, we seem to be pretty proficient in that arena. We hurt others and we betray our values. We accumulate all sorts of bad baggage such as guilt, low self-worth, self-loathing, fear, rage, and depression. Depression is part of addiction. My own categorization of depression includes situational depression, drug-induced depression, and chemical imbalance depression. Let me explain.

Situational Depression: Every addict has a pile of adverse consequences, and sooner or later he or she gets buried under them and sees no way out. If you just lost your car, your spouse, your kids, and your residence, and you are sitting in a jail cell for possession of illegal substances or your third DUI, you are going to be depressed. You have put yourself in a crappy situation, and you're supposed to be depressed. As a matter of fact, with all this going on it would be abnormal not to be depressed. If you get into recovery, get your family back, get your finances straight, and resolve your legal issues, that depression should lift.

Drug-Induced Depression: The official name of this type of depression is Substance-Induced Mood Disorder. If you are coming down after a methamphetamine binge and have burned your nerve endings to a crisp (figuratively), you are in for a rebound, or drug-induced depression. If you are loaded up on alcohol and wallowing in self-pity, you will get depressed. If you anesthetized your brain with opiates long enough, you may have given yourself a condition called anhedonia. Anhedonia means you are "just numbed out" and nothing makes you happy. This may be due to the overload drugs have put on the reward center in your brain. That reward center is the nucleus accumbens or NA. Once you get some recovery time, your NA should begin healing, and this type of depression should lift. Notice I said recovery time not dry time.

Chemical Imbalance Depression: This type of depression is just that, a neurochemical imbalance. You may be been genetically vulnerable to developing this type of depression which of course means depression may run in your family. Even if you enter recovery, you still carry the depression, and you need treatment for it. You may have a Major Depressive Disorder, or a Bipolar Disorder. As an aside, Bill Wilson suffered from severe depressive episodes even after he co-founded Alcoholics Anonymous and was sober for years. Regrettably, he did not have the benefit of today's medications. You do.

Observably in addiction, all of these types of depression can occur, and they can all occur at the same time. These are not clear-cut categories. Indeed, there is usually overlap. Actually, I use these categories for a point of reference when discussing depression with my addict patients. Unless there is a clear diagnosis of depression, I suggest waiting a few weeks before committing someone to a medication course that will go on for months.

Antidepressant medications are considered mood elevators only to the extent that they allow your brain chemicals and receptors to function normally. If the type or level of depression present requires medical treatment, we will try to match the medication to the predominant symptom. For instance, if you have a depression associated with anxiety, the best choice would be an antidepressant with some anti-anxiety effects. There are some antidepressant medications that are more "energizing" than others. Such medications would be a first choice if you are depressed and have fatigue. Other types of antidepressant medications have proven to be better for depression associated with Post Traumatic Stress Disorders. In some patients, an antidepressant may be combined with a mood stabilizer.

Genetic testing can help point us to the best drug for an individual. This technology has advanced to the point that we can take a genetic swab from your mouth and send it off to find out what medication might work best you. This technology does have a place in medication choices. This genetic guidance, although refined, is really nothing new. I was trained to ask what medications work for any depressed family member you might have and then recommend that same medication to you. The chances are what worked for a family member will work for you. It is not foolproof, and like anything else, genetic testing is a tool, not an answer.

There is one caveat applicable to addicts, and that is the fact that antidepressants do not work overnight. They take time to work. It may take weeks for an antidepressant to kick in. Since addicts like immediate results, they may decide the medication is useless and abandon taking it.

I really do have people come into my office the very next day after taking an antidepressant to tell me that they do not feel any better yet and maybe we should try something else. This occurs even though I have explained how long the medication takes to start working prior to prescribing it. I am not irritated or surprised when this happens because I know that patience is not the strongest character trait in addiction.

Even with genetic testing, it may be necessary to try different antidepressants until one antidepressant works or until we find a combination of medications that is effective. Once the need for an antidepressant is established, and we find one that works, you can expect to be on it for at least six months. The critical variable here is that you comply with treatment and take it as prescribed.
So what happens after six months?

The six-month mark is not an automatic thing. That six-month mark is based on several variables. If you are an addict in recovery, your brain will have undergone some healing within that six-month period. During that time of sobriety, your social situation tends to improve, and there may be less situational depression. Therefore, the actual time you should be taking the medication depends on how you are doing and feeling. If your depression has lifted and you want to get off the medication, we can discuss tapering off. We do this slowly and monitor your mood as we taper the medication dosage downward.

If your depression has cleared and stays that way as we taper you off, you have no need to continue it. If your depression returns as we are tapering your dose down, we can stabilize the dose and consider trying to decrease it again in another six months. Remember, these medications are not altering your mood, they are helping you repair or compensate for neurological dysfunction or damage due to use of addictive substances.

Do not do discontinue medications on your own. Work with your healthcare provider, who is prescribing the medication and your therapist and keep your sponsor apprised of what is going on. If you are tapering off an antidepressant, you might ask your sponsor to be on the lookout for any mood changes. I am not suggesting in any way that your sponsor should be treating you or giving out medical advice. Your family also needs to be aware of what is going on.

Treatment requires an individualized treatment plan that you help create. As addicts, we collect all sorts of negative emotions. Some unique issues are pathological grief, guilt about irreparable damage done to others, all sorts of PTSD issues, brain damage from automobile crashes, complex relationship issues, etc. The point here is that "one size does not fit all" nor does one medication fit all depressions. Of course, if you relapse, all this is moot because everything goes to hell in a hand basket with relapse.

Pathological Grief: Mourning is the term given to the expected sadness that accompanies a significant loss such as the death of a loved one. Mourning is a painful process of cascading negative emotional states. The process ultimately allows the person experiencing the loss to move forward with his or her life. Mourning is an individualized process that is molded by numerous variables such as culture, social expectations, significance of the loss, unexpected or untimely death, individual emotional resilience, and a host of other variables beyond the scope of this conversation. While loss and grief can be relapse triggers for a recovering addict, our focus here is on pathological grief as a variable of active addiction. The person experiencing pathological grief can be envisioned as being stuck in the grief process. They often exhibit guilt and shame related to the death of the loved one. The may have misdirected hostility towards self, others, and/or God. Subsequently, they may continue to addictively use mood-altering substances. Drinking and drugging can impair the ability to progress through the normal grief process. Indeed, some addicts have to grieve giving up the grief in order to recover. It is a complex process that requires honesty, openness, and willingness. Many years ago, I was sitting in a group process, and this very issue was being addressed.

> *Trent was teary eyed as he related to the group that he drank because he could not get over his mother's death. She had died sixteen years ago, and he was still slugging down a fifth of vodka a day behind it. Some of the people in group were trying to console him and give him suggestions on how to get through the grief process and sharing their experiences about the loss of a loved one. A lot of the*

group members were sympathizing with Trent who was 47 years old at the time. All this stopped rather abruptly when the counselor injected a different viewpoint.

"If you loved your mother so much, you have a crappy way of showing it. You are using the tragedy of her death to stay drunk and dishonor her. You disgust me." Counselor Joe.

You could have heard a pin drop in that room.

"If you want to get through this, I will help you. But if you want to stay a victim and use your poor dead mother as your reason for being a drunk, this is probably not the place for you. Sitting on that pity pot and trying to make everyone feel sorry for you is going to kill you." Counselor Joe.

Wow! Like I said this was a long time ago when confrontation "therapy" was the standard. I expected him to jump up, spit out some profanities, and blow out of treatment. He did storm out of group, but he did not leave treatment. He came back after group was over and had a one to one session with the counselor. The counselor gave him some assignments, and he started working on them. Trent actually ended up coming back and apologizing to the group later for being manipulative. He even asked the group not to enable his self-pity. That took a lot of courage.

In addition to getting into recovery and AA, he did some alcohol-free grief counseling, and from what I understand, he is still sober.

In this day and age, most programs would probably not be so confrontational (at least not my programs), but we would make it clear to Trent that as long as he was drinking, he would not make any progress with grief resolution. We would establish boundaries and not play into his "self-pity." Once he was dry, we would help him go through the grief process and provide him with the necessary insight, tools, techniques, and support to get some resolution and abandon his victim role. His task would not have been any easier, but he would receive input within the motivational therapy paradigm which he might find more palatable. The motivational model seems to decrease the risk of the person becoming so defensive that he or she rejects treatment and resumes self-destructive behaviors. People support what they help create.

Trent was locked into rigid thinking and rigid emotions. He really had little insight into that rigidity, but everyone around him with any wherewithal could see it. Rigidity resists change, and misery was as rigidly normal for him as relief drinking was. You may recall that one of the things wrong with an alcoholic brain is that it does not know what is wrong with it. Over the years I have witnessed some patients respond (i.e., change their behaviors) after being through a "shame-based" program. I have also seen patients and families harmed by that approach. I do not condone this type of treatment, but there are some therapists who still embrace it.

There are many questions about the shame-based approach. Did Trent get sober because of that treatment experience or in spite of it? Would another approach have produced the same or better result? Was the whole tone of his treatment "heavy confrontation of his denial"? What are the outcome studies for this type of "tear down" and "build up" therapy? As you may also recall, outcome studies are lacking for many programs. There are a variety of reasons for that lack, and there is still no universal standard to define treatment.

A brief history of the evolution of the Substance Abuse Counseling Profession and the field of Addiction Medicine as a whole may help put some of these issues into perspective.

Historically, organized medicine has lagged behind when it comes to treating the brain disease of addictions. In was not until 1956, 21 years after Bill Wilson and Bob Smith founded Alcoholics Anonymous, that the American Medical Association (AMA) classified alcoholism as a disease. This should not be misinterpreted as a period of great medical enlightenment for the disease of addiction but it was a start. Notice the AMA classified **alcoholism** as a disease, but it did not classify drug addiction as a disease.

This separatist attitude between alcoholism and drug addiction was reflected in the "treatment community" as well. Many people involved in the treatment of alcoholism considered drug addiction a sort of "other entity." On a personal note, when I started going to AA in the late 1970s, I was politely told not to mention my drug addiction in an AA meeting and to stick to alcoholism as a topic. It was even announced at the beginning of the meeting.

> *"We do not talk about drug addiction here. We talk about alcoholism. If you start talking about drug addiction, we may ask you to leave."*

It was not until the 1980s that the integration of treatment for alcoholism and drug addictions became acceptable as the norm. Moreover it was not until 1987 that the AMA termed addiction a disease. Just to put that date into context, Narcotics Anonymous was founded in 1953!

Organized medicine lagged behind and left a deadly destructive void in the delivery of care for addicts and alcoholics who sorely needed treatment. The void was filled by addiction counselors.

In those "old days" a counselor was often someone who was in recovery, had a year or two of sobriety, did a year or so on-the-job training, and was dubbed a counselor. They were referred to as "para-professionals" in some of the literature of the time. They were often locked into their own rigid approaches that were based upon their own personal journeys into sobriety. A grass roots movement evolved to get addiction counselors credentialed. Organizations were established at local and national levels to improve the standards of the counseling field. It worked. This has been a "grandfathering" process, and most qualified therapists today have Masters Level Degrees.

In 1988, the American Medical Society of Addiction Medicine was admitted into the American Medical Society.

We have come a long way.

Bipolar and Substance Use Disorder

The term Bipolar Disorder actually refers to a spectrum of mental illnesses characterized by significant mood swings. The classical manic depressive disorder is referred to as Bipolar I Disorder. To make such a diagnosis, the patient must have a history of at least one "manic" episode that lasts for at least a week. During a manic phase, the person is very hyperactive and obviously impaired.

This mother's description of her 21-year-old son's first manic episode illustrates some of the symptoms of mania.

*"It was scary. Bernie started getting **irritable** for a few days then he started **staying up all night** and walking the floors. He would **jump from one topic to another.** As a matter of fact, he was **talking so fast** that I couldn't get in a word edgewise. He said he was feeling full of energy and his <u>thoughts were racing</u> through his head. I found out later he was **drinking a half fifth** of whiskey at night trying to get to sleep. Then he got it into his mind that **he could predict** the winning numbers on the roulette wheel at the casino. I was shocked at this because we don't approve of gambling in our family. Then again, we do not approve of drinking either. But I was even more shocked when I got a call that he had been arrested for <u>a</u>**ttacking someone** at the casino boat. They said he was in there trying to get strange women to **have sex** with him and then he decided the casino was cheating him. It was a real mess. We got him to a psychiatric hospital, and they said his drug screen showed "synthetic marijuana." They say that may have triggered this whole thing. My sister is Bipolar so it **runs in the family.** Anyway, the hospital kept him a few weeks and he leveled out. He is back home now but he is getting more and more **depressed."***

Bipolar II Disorder is a less intense form of the disease and the mood swings are not as extreme. The hypomanic person has lots of energy and may seem "hyper" and "bubbly." The person may not sleep much, may talk rapidly, may jump from topic to topic, have some rapid thoughts, be easily distractible, exhibit risk-taking behaviors, and act impulsively. Some Bipolar II patients really enjoy the hypomanic state and may use drugs in an effort to stay there. This impaired decision tends to have a poor outcome. The downward cycle into depression, although usually not as severe as that experienced with the Bipolar I variety, can be debilitating.

Another variation of Bipolar Disorder is the "Mixed State" in which there is a mixture of mania as well as depression. This is really a mixed bag of symptoms including depression, agitation, insomnia, anxiety, rapid mood changes, and increased risk for suicide. This "mixed state" is not a simple, straightforward diagnosis, and it can be even more confusing in someone using alcohol and drugs.

Most bipolar patients, if not adequately treated, live in a depressed state most of the time. Indeed, without proper treatment, Bipolar II patients may live in a state of depression seventy percent of their lifetimes. As a matter of fact, twenty percent of patients who see a doctor for depression are actually bipolar. Differentiating the unipolar from the bipolar patient has major therapeutic implications. For one thing, antidepressants are the mainstay medical treatment for unipolar depression, but they may actually trigger a manic episode in the bipolar patient who presents with depression.

Manic episodes lead to more manic episodes. More episodes may result in brain cell degeneration. Not surprisingly, glutamate may play a role in this brain-damaging effect. There is a medication by the name of memantine that is getting a lot of interest from researchers. It is used in the treatment of Alzheimer's and other dementia. It may be protective during mania and can be added to the medication treatment regimen for a bipolar patient. Memantine decreases glutamate's excitoxoic effect and may thereby protect brain cells and cognitive function in the bipolar patient.

People who suffer with Bipolar Disorders have a forty percent chance of also having a substance use disorder. Of special note is the risk factor that inadequately treated alcohol withdrawal may trigger a manic episode. The coexistence of addiction and a bipolar disorder of any type results in higher relapse rates for both disorders and a higher risk for suicide than for either disorder alone.

As noted above, some bipolar patients self-medicate to try and maintain their hypomanic state. They do this with drugs like amphetamines or cocaine which in turn fuel paranoia. When the dual-diagnosed person stops taking the amphetamine or cocaine, the depressive rebound can be very pronounced.

During the depressive phase of a bipolar disorder, it is not uncommon to see an increase in benzodiazepine abuse in the person who also has a Substance Use Disorder. I am not sure why this happens, but this is a clinical pearl worth knowing because the person may become physically dependent on the benzodiazepines while trying to self-medicate the depression spiral of his or her Bipolar Disorder. Of course, you do not have to be Bipolar to self-medicate depression inappropriately. There is also a high risk of benzodiazepine abuse in a person suffering from a Major Depressive Disorder.

There are other signs that a person might be at increased risk for developing a Bipolar Disorder. Young people at risk for Bipolar Disorder have a diminished subjective experience with alcohol. This means that if they drink alcohol, they do not feel as drunk as a peer without the risk of Bipolar Disorder. Therefore, they need to drink more to get a feeling of intoxication. Accordingly, if you are a clinician taking a drug history on a patient and find a high tolerance to ethanol, you might be on the alert for any additional clues for the development of a Bipolar Disorder. Of course high tolerance to alcoholic in a young person is not diagnostic of Bipolar Disorder. Indeed, it may just be a clue to alcohol dependency.

Treatment: As with any chronic relapsing disorder, treatment and monitoring should continue indefinitely. The medications of choice for Bipolar Disorders are the mood stabilizers and antipsychotics. These include:

- **Mood Stabilizers:**
  - Lithium
  - Carbamazepine (Tegretol)
  - Valproic acid or divalproex (Depakote)
  - Lamotrigine (Lamictal)
  - Oxcarbazeoine (Trileptal)
  - Topitamate (Topomax)
- **Atypical Antipsychotics:**
  - Apripiprazole (Abilify)
  - Olanzapine (Zyprexa)
  - Quetiapine (Seroquel)
  - Risperidone (Risperdal)
  - Ziprasidone (Geodon)
  - Lurasidone (Latuda)

As mentioned earlier, pregnancy is a particularly vulnerable time for mood swings in Bipolar Disorders. These medications can have significant adverse effects on the fetus which complicates the treatment of Bipolar Disorders during pregnancy.

Antidepressants: Prescribing antidepressants for Bipolar Disorders is controversial at best. It is very ill advised to prescribe an antidepressant alone to a bipolar patient as this may cause rapid cycling. The antidepressants that are thought to have the least potential to cause cycling are Wellbutrin (bupropion) and Paxil (paroxetine). The atypical antipsychotic, Latuda, is approved for treatment of Bipolar Depression. I do not prescribe any antidepressant as monotherapy for a bipolar patient, but I often see patients show up in my practice who tell me they are Bipolar yet are on antidepressants without the benefit of mood stabilizers. Take Lori Beth for example:

She is a 26-year-old female who presents for detoxification from alcohol, IV opioids (roxy and heroin), and benzodiazepines (Xanax and Klonopin). She also smokes marijuana but feels this is not an issue. She smokes a pack of cigarettes a day and has no intent of quitting. Every now and then she will use cocaine IV. During the course of my interview, she tells me she has a diagnosis of Bipolar Disorder. When I asked her about how this diagnosis came to be, she related this series of events.

"I tried to kill myself when I was 21 years old, and I ended up in the psych hospital. I was drunk. I do not remember much of it. I was still in a fog when some young doctor asked me all sorts of questions. Like why was I drinking? I told him because I was wired up and needed to come down. Of course, I lied about how much cocaine I used. I told him there must have been some in the blunt we smoked. He actually believed that crap. He asked about my moods, and I told him they were up and down. He told me I was Bipolar and put me on a bunch of drugs that really zonked me out. As soon as I got

out of there, I stopped most of them, but I stayed on the Effexor in the morning because it seemed to help a little. Later, some other doctor gave me Trazodone 300 mg to take a night. And then another one gave me some Remeron to take at night. Hell, I was not sleeping because the dope gives me energy. But it worked out. Whenever I would get really messed up and would act all stupid, my mom would say it was due to the Bipolar. I got away with all kinds of crap behind the 'Bipolar made me do it' excuse. Of course, that generally meant a trip to the funny farm, but it beats being thrown out on the streets or going to jail. When I would go in,

I would have a diagnosis of Bipolar and it stuck. I will tell you right now, I am not taking any Depakote or any crazy pills. I used to cheek them in the nut house. Do I think I am Bipolar? No. I read up about Bipolar, and I damn sure do not have that problem, but I do need my home meds to sleep while I am here."

It is difficult to figure out what is really going on with Lori Beth. I doubt she has Bipolar Disorder, but she has carried that label for at least five years. She may have a Substance Induced Mood Disorder. She may have depression. She may have a Personality Disorder. I am sure of only two things. If she has a Bipolar Disorder, her medication regimen is not appropriate and speaks against a diagnosis of Bipolar Disorder. The only other thing I am certain about is that she is an addict, and that is her primary presenting problem. There is no way to make any other legitimate diagnosis until she is sober for a while.

PERSONALITY DISORDERS

There are three personality disorders that present themselves with some regularity in my patient population. These are Borderline Personality Disorder, Narcissistic Personality Disorder, and Sociopathic Personality Disorder.

> *"I have been to a psych hospital before because they thought I was **trying to kill myself**. All I did was cut my wrist. See here is that scar. I did it after I caught my boyfriend with someone else. I am a **Borderline Personality,** so I do things like that. I get **real impulsive** and I have **temper outbursts**. I like to run with the bad boys because I am one of the bad girls. Drugs are fun for me, but I do not want to go back to jail, so here I am."*

> *"I got busted and I cussed the cop out. She was a real bitch to me anyway. Then they looked in my car, and I had some drugs and some stuff I stole from **my other ex-boyfriend**. I really did not want his stuff, I just did it to get even with him. I keyed his car too. They had me on suicide watch in jail because I beat my fist against the wall."* Gloria is a 23 year old admitted for methamphetamine addiction. She has been in jail for two weeks because her parents would not bail her out unless she agreed to treatment.

Gloria may very well suffer from Borderline Personality Disorder, but just like Lori Beth in our prior scenario, her diagnosis needs to be verified. The reason I say this is because the brain disease of addiction is also known to be a great imposter. It is not shocking news to anyone that addicts lie about their addictions. When they show up at an emergency department with psychotic symptoms and lie about the fact they just smokes three bowls of "MoJo" (synthetic marijuana) and the drug screen is negative (because synthetic marijuana is not detected on a routine drug screen), they get labeled as "crazy" or psychotic. Moreover if they keep lying, they may end up on all sorts of medications for psychiatric illnesses they do not have.

There are real dangers in putting a label on someone and tagging them as a personality disorder. Labels have lasting implications. By definition, you cannot change a personality disorder. Your personality is who you are. At best you can help the person learn acceptable behaviors. As the person ages, the personality disorder may mellow somewhat, but they have usually left behind a trail of damage and destruction in their paths.

Labels have other dangers. A label can become a self-fulfilling prophecy. I have treated patients who research their "diagnosis" and then try to live up to it. They also project it as a facade to excuse their behaviors. A label can also "explain" to the person why they do what they do, but it can be the wrong explanation if the diagnosis is wrong. Indeed, it can detract from the need to address their addictive brain disease. Like Gloria said:

> "I am a Borderline Personality, so I do things like that."

This type of self-talk can doom Gloria to repeat and act out her behaviors and continue her active addiction ad infinitum.

Another danger of having a personality disorder label is that therapists may "pigeon hole" her with expectations as to how she will respond to treatment. These expectations can actually promote Gloria to act out. Some therapists actually exclude people with personality disorder, from becoming patients in their practices.

Traits: There is another somewhat confusing labeling issue worth mentioning in relation to diagnosing personality disorders. The person may not fulfill the diagnosis of a personality disorder but may have some of the traits of the disorder. Drug addicts exhibit all sorts of destructive and socially unacceptable traits as they violate their values to keep their addictions going. They lie, cheat, steal, hide, have outbursts, blame others, think the world should accommodate them, feel entitled, and are destructive to self and others. In short, they exhibit personality disorder traits. When they get into recovery these behaviors remit, and they no longer fulfill the criteria for having these traits. That is a good thing.

However, those same behaviors can show up on psychological testing as being "disorders." This is another reason I do not like to make a diagnosis of anything other than Substance Use Disorder in addicted patients for at least a month after acute detox and ongoing treatment unless there is strong clinical evidence that they have a co-existing disorder that must be addressed. Along that same line of reasoning, I may challenge a pre-existing diagnosis if the evidence does not support that diagnosis the addict walks through the door with.

Having said all that, personality disorders exist and if Gloria does have a Borderline Personality Disorder, as well as addiction, there are some specific therapeutic measures that can be employed to help her. She will require long-term care with clear-cut expectations and consequences. Even if she has a personality disorder, she can learn to deal with it and not be a victim of it.

We are going to explore the personality disorders not infrequently encountered in people also having addictive brains. There is one caveat to mention before we have a look at these specific disorders. These disorders tend to overlap in some patients, and we too want to avoid the "pigeon hole" trap.

Borderline Personality Disorder: This entity tends to occur more in females, so we will continue to cite Gloria as our example. She exhibits three main areas of dysfunction. Her relationships with others are often volatile or even explosive at times. She tends to idolize a person one week and demonize him or her the next week. She has sort of an all-or-none viewpoint about people. Watch out for whirlwind romances. If you are the recipient of Gloria's idealized affection and seductions, you may feel flattered, but as time goes on and you are subjected to her intense fears of abandonment, you may try to draw away. At that point you become devalued and may become the recipient of some degree of wrath. The relationship tends to get very rocky when you are not able to meet her emotional needs. Gloria may target you with jealous tirades because she has significant fear of abandonment. She may feel the need to retaliate for your real or imagined treason in the relationship. Her moods tend to swing quickly and dramatically. She often complains of feeling empty and anxious and does things just to compensate for those feelings. Those things she does to compensate may include destructive behaviors such as excessive spending, binging on alcohol, binging on drugs, self-mutilation, and/or stealing. When she gets into such trouble, she may end up in treatment. It may not be her first time there. Her behaviors may look manic in nature, and it may be difficult to make an accurate diagnosis until she clears from the chemicals.

Gloria may have some dysfunction in her amygdala and her prefrontal cortex. We talked about these parts of the brain before. Since the amygdala is the fight or flight brain area, her overactive amygdale may account in part to her severe fear of rejection. We also know the prefrontal cortex (PFC) is where our decision making is regulated. If Gloria has an underactive PFC, she is going to have inappropriate outbursts and poor impulse control. This may put her in dangerous situations that ultimately result in all sort of adverse consequences such as physical abuse, incarceration, drug overdose, suicide attempts, and even suicide.

Treatment for Borderline Personality Disorder requires consistency on the part of the therapist. There are some anticonvulsant medications that can help stabilize Gloria's mood and decrease her angry outbursts. Antipsychotic medications may also be of some benefit. However, antidepressants may not offer much value for a personality disorder per se. Gloria's treatment plan will have emphasis on recovery from her addiction and stabilization of her Borderline Personality Disorder. She will require long term care for both. There are "sober living houses" that can be included in her ongoing treatment plan. She requires accountability, consistency, stability, boundaries, and monitoring.

Self-Harm, for our clinical purposes, is defined as self-injury without suicidal intent. Being a Borderline Personality Disorder is a risk factor for self-harm but so are child trauma, child abuse, and/or sexual trauma. The majority of self-harmers are females. Self-harm may manifest as self-cutting, scratching, self-hitting, hitting walls, and/or burning one's self. For some females, multiple piercing and tattoos are a form of self-harm.

> Jenna has multiple tattoos and multiple piercings in various places on her body. Some of her tats are "homemade." She is being treated today for twenty some odd superficial abrasions to her right inner thigh. She cut herself with a razor blade. She has old scars on her arms and legs from previous similar

behaviors. There are a couple of healed cigarette burns on the left forearm.

"I needed some relief, so I cut myself. You know? The pain lets me know I am still alive and not some numbed out lump of meat. You know? That is one of the reasons I like tattoos; they hurt. Sometimes cutting makes me feel good, like dope. You know? I hate it when people think I am doing it because I'm suicidal. You know? I am not suicidal. I just get to where I want to cut myself. You know?"

Narcissistic Personality Disorder: The name origin of this disorder is most descriptive. According to ancient Greek mythology, Narcissus was a beautiful hunter who fell in love with his own reflection. So what, right? I mean you can go to the local muscle gym and see that phenomenon in action. The difference is that Narcissus was so enthralled by his own beautiful reflection that he could not tear himself away from it and died admiring himself. That, my friends, is definitely self-love run riot. Here's an example of narcissism:

"People are jealous of me because of who I am and how I look. I am just a natural leader and other people are attracted to me because of it. I have always been good at everything I do. Not many 23-year-old guys are making four hundred bucks a day selling Ecstasy. Right? My customers know I have a quality product. That's why they come to me. I would never have gotten caught except for some jealous rat turning me in. I am way too smart for that. I can have any woman I want, but I get bored with them pretty quickly. I have a couple of kids out there, but their mothers take care of them. I give them some money when they need it. I do not need to be here, but I have to do this for the courts. My dad has a lawyer fixing all this. What I want is to complete this program and get my treatment

certificate. I do not need to be here as long as these other people. I can knock this out in a couple of weeks if you guys let me do it my way. Then I can get back in college. I may go into psychology." Mac is a 23-year-old ecstasy dealer. This is his fourth treatment center since age 19.

Mac is obviously self-centered and expects the universe to revolve around him. He feels others owe him simply because of who he is. He projects himself as arrogant and self-assured. He has no remorse for taking advantage of others because they exist to serve him and his needs. He has the world by the tail. Or does he? Mac cannot stand to have anyone criticize him. When he does get criticism, it worries him and he cannot let it go. He may seek out others to shore up his self-esteem by having them reassure him that he is perfect. He will belittle and discount any criticism because in reality he has a fragile self-esteem and a great deal of inner shame.

Few people with normal self-esteem will tolerate being around someone with this sort of personality disorder. They view Mac as a selfish, boring braggart with only one interest, himself. Mac may even start to believe his own outlandish lies and then wonder why people talk about him behind his back. Mac may also find that constantly admiring his reflection can be a very lonely obsession.

If you are wondering what it might be like to marry a narcissist, you have only to read the Greek myth about the woman (wood nymph) who was madly in love with Narcissus. Her name was Echo. Her love was not returned because Narcissus loved only Narcissus. His cruel rejection was devastating to the point that she watched helplessly as he died by the reflecting pool admiring himself. Sickened by grief, her physical form faded away and her bones became rocks. All that remained was her voice, and it could only repeat the last things she heard. She became an Echo.

Antisocial Personality Disorder: This is the person who has no regard for right or wrong. They lie, cheat, steal, manipulate, abuse, exploit, bully, and have no remorse for doing so. They tend to have all sorts of legal problems, both criminal and civil. You can forget child support from them because they lack empathy for anyone including their kids. These people can be charismatic and attract other into their web of deceit. The jails are full of these types. They often have a history of being cruel, defiant and oppositional during childhood. Stay away from these people.

Clusters- Often times in the clinical world, we use the word cluster to describe personality characteristic that are pathological. We noted earlier that there may be some overlap in personality disorders. There are three broad clusters.

Cluster A includes the people who are usually described by those who know them as eccentric or odd when being politically correct. They are often described as "weird" when their names come up at family gatherings. (Gatherings they usually do not attend for a variety of reasons.) This group includes paranoid personality disordered people who never forget a real or imagined insult or slight. Not only do they hold grudges forever, they may be prone to lawsuits. Many times they are loners. This is no surprise. If they think everyone is out to get them why on earth would they want to be around anyone? At one end of this cluster spectrum are those who have odd beliefs and unique experiences such as seeing bizarre nondescript things. These folks are sort of on the fringe of being schizophrenic. Some of these folks are so paranoid that they feel a pre-emptive attack is justified on others. Those of you my age might remember Theodore (Ted) Kaczynski, better known as the "Unabomber." He lived a hermit's existence in a cabin in Montana and mailed bombs out to people from 1978 to 1995. He seems to fit the Type A Schizotypal Diagnosis.

At any rate, from a clinical perspective, the Cluster A folks are very difficult to engage in treatment.

Cluster B is where our girl Gloria would fit in. These people tend to have poor impulse control. In addition to the borderline, this cluster also includes the "Histrionic." The histrionics are the "drama queens." Things really get fired up when you have several of these residing in the same treatment cabin. They like the spotlight, and they want to be the center of attention. Just like the Borderline, they are usually female and can be very seductive, flighty, and erratic. They do not like being alone. Interestingly, they are quite vulnerable to being controlled by the opinions of others and therefore vulnerable to co-dependency. The Narcissist falls into this cluster as does the Antisocial.

From a clinical perspective, the therapist needs to establish strong boundaries and expectations. The Cluster B folks are going to challenge those boundaries and will probably exhibit emotional dysregulation with outbursts and the like.

Cluster C consists of people who are driven by fear and anxiety. Many of these people simply miss out on life and/or avoid it altogether. Hence they are labeled as having Avoidant Personality Disorders. They avoid social events and social interactions. They are fearful that they will embarrass themselves in public. They have a very poor self-image and low self-worth.

Another group of this Cluster C category includes those with a Dependent Personality Disorder. This personality disorder is just what it sounds like. These people need someone to tell them what to do. They are easily manipulated and pushed around. They cling to others and are "door mats'.

The other part of Cluster C is composed of the people with an Obsessive-Compulsive Personality Disorder. These are the people who "go by the book." They are often rigid in their approach to life. They are given to perfectionism so they are always anxious since perfectionism is a myth. They may have difficulty delegating to others. They may have obsessions such as the need to keep everything germ free. They may have compulsive rituals such as checking to see if the door is locked 27 times.

Cluster C treatment includes Cognitive Behavioral Therapy techniques.

PAIN AND ADDICTION

Physical pain falls into two broad categories: acute pain and chronic pain. Addicts often have pain issues for a variety of reasons. We fall down, walk into furniture, get into fights, wreck vehicles, etc. Plus, when we are in an active addiction, we tend not to take care of ourselves and get things like tooth abscesses. Then when we get sober, we decide to deal with all of these problems at once. As noted earlier, patience is not usually our strong suit. There are also those unfortunates who have chronic pain and have fallen into the trap of taking escalating doses of opiate medication and/or benzodiazepines to the point of becoming addicted.

I think this is a good time to talk about the difference between physical dependency and addiction. Anyone who takes opiates on a regular basis for one or two weeks is going to have some level of physical dependency. We know the brain alters itself to deal with opiates coming in from outside the body (via skin, mouth, nose, lung, vein, or other route).

Physical dependency in and of itself does not fulfill the diagnostic criteria of addiction. For dependency to rise to the level of addiction, there must be loss of control over taking the substance, need to increase the dosage, and continued use despite the fact that negative consequences are piling up due to that usage.

Anyone can become physically dependent on an addictive drug. To prove that fact, we can do a little "virtual" experiment.

> *If one hundred randomly selected people would let me put an IV into their arms and push escalating doses of morphine into them for two weeks, I would have one hundred opiate dependent people on my*

hands. Then, let us say I stop all IV's and, therefore, all morphine abruptly. I now have one hundred people in a state of opiate withdrawal. They all have the sweats and aches and chills and anxiety and diarrhea and yawning – all of it.

Then after they go through all that, I tell them the experiment was flawed and we have to repeat it. Eight-five to ninety of the participants would refuse me and probably call me unkind names, but ten to fifteen of them would be ready and willing to repeat it right away. Those are the ones who liked the drug effect so much they will readily do it again despite knowing how bad the detox will be after two weeks. These are the people who have "the addiction circuits" and those addictive circuits have been activated. These are the addicts. The people who do not have the addictive circuits think those who have addictive circuits are crazy because they are volunteering to do it again.

This outcome is not surprising because between ten to fifteen percent of the current population has or will have a substance use disorder. For our purposes, we will use a mean of thirteen percent. Our virtual experiment really was not flawed at all. The goal was to discover how many addicts we would discover in one hundred randomly chosen subjects. We ended up with eighty-seven opiate-dependent non-addicts and thirteen opiate-dependent addicts. This was an expected outcome.

Of course, we would never condone such an unethical, dangerous experiment in the first place. Why would we? There is no need for such a research project because this scenario is going on every day in the USA. If you have moderate to severe pain, there is a high likelihood that an opiate will be prescribed to you. If you are one of the thirteen percent prone to addiction, you may end up in trouble.

Indeed, the relatively liberal opioid prescribing practices in the USA account for the fact that we Americans ingest ninety-nine percent of the hydrocodone produced in the WORLD!

Acute Pain and the Recovering Addict

What if I have to take pain medication that is addictive?
This is every recovering person's concern. If you are an addict and do not have this concern, then you do not have a grasp on the concept of the brain disease of addiction. What's an addict to do? Several things. Here is an example.

Karen is a 28-year-old female who completed her initial treatment about six months ago. As part of her recovery plan, she decided to start getting in shape by bicycling. She will readily admit that one of her character traits is that she does nothing in moderation. After one week of biking she decided to bike down some steps at LSU. After all, she just saw two other girls do it. She now finds herself in the emergency room and in a great deal of pain. An x-ray reveals a fracture of her lower leg that will require corrective surgery but for right now, it requires stabilization. Historically, Karen's drug of choice is oxycodone.

She is in great pain but she is also worried about relapsing as her addiction almost cost her everything. Karen is in the midst of a dangerous dilemma, but she has several things going in her favor. Karen has been attending AA on a regular basis and has established a home group. She also has a sponsor with some long-term sobriety from opiate addiction. In keeping with her written "Relapse Prevention Plan" which she developed in treatment, her sponsor has already been notified of Karen's situation and is on her way up to the emergency room.

Karen has confided in the ER doctor that she is in recovery. The doctor confided that his mother is also in recovery and assures Karen that he will treat her pain adequately but will try to "keep her out of trouble." As Karen is rolled into the operating room for bone stabilization, she is grateful that her support network is there for her. Karen will require postoperative medication and this will be controlled by her mother. Karen will keep in close contact with her sponsor and other people in her home group. She will notify her addictionologist of the situation. She is in a high-risk situation for relapse and refuses to be a victim. Karen knows the importance of keeping those healthy brain circuits working by continuing to work her recovery program and utilizing her support network.

In the event that you are in recovery and you require a mood-altering substance, you should have a Relapse Prevention Plan in place. Notify all healthcare providers of your diagnosis. Put aside the fear that "they will not give me enough pain medication if they know I am an addict." For one thing you are not an addict. You are a person in recovery, and most healthcare providers respect that. Activate your support system. Have a trusted third party to be in charge of your medication. Keep working your program even if you cannot get out to meetings. Let your addictionologist know what is going on. Do not become a victim of yourself.

Chronic Pain and the Recovering Addict

Chronic pain is a whole different situation than that of acute pain. The pain mechanisms are different and treatment is different. Opiates can actually make the pain worse over the long haul.

Chronic pain is associated with multiple problems. One problem with chronic pain is the risk of "deconditioning" of muscles, bones, and joints. Identifying one's self as a "pain patient" may set up a self-fulfilling prophecy of being a victim. Depression and chronic pain go hand-in-hand for a lot of folks. Indeed, the person with chronic pain may be more prone to develop a major depressive disorder.

Then there is the whole realm of "secondary gain." Secondary gain is getting some reward for having chronic pain. These rewards can come in all sorts of ways:
- The ability to get drugs because of pain
- Financial gain
- Keeping family members hostage through their feelings of sympathy, undeserved loyalty, and even guilt

I am not saying every addict with chronic pain is seeking secondary gain. What I am saying is that these are things that must be considered in treatment.

Here is an example of "secondary gain" by a family member:

Mrs. Shirley Castile entered treatment at the insistence of her daughter, Carolyn. Mrs. Castile (Shirley) sustained a severe work-related injury to her lower back twelve years ago. She lives with her daughter who has three young children. Carolyn's husband has been "out of the picture" for several years. Shirley has continued to increase her use of prescription opiates to the point that she has been buying them from "friends" she met at the pain clinic. Historically, her role in the family has been to take care of the kids while Carolyn works outside the home. Of course, her disability check is factored into the household budget.

Shirley is also addicted to Xanax which was prescribed for her anxiety and muscle spasms. Her addiction has gotten to the point where she passes out on the couch, and the kids run free. One of the children was recently injured in a preventable home accident, and Carolyn blames her mother who is full of guilt about it all. "That was the last straw."

During the course of treatment, Shirley has regained much of her self-worth and self-confidence. Her pain has decreased with non-opiate treatment. One of her problems was hyperalgesia, which means the opiates were actually causing her to feel more pain. Shirley has been walking and going to the gym and tells me, "The pain is still there but I can live with it." She shares in a family session that she is still young enough to have a career and a job.

When those words come out of Shirley's mouth, you can hear the proverbial pin drop. Carolyn is "taken aback." Carolyn's face looks frozen in a state of panic and she blurts out, "You can't do that. We need that disability check. What if you get off disability and relapse? That would be the end of us. Momma! Think about what you are saying. That would be a selfish thing to do to us."

It seems that Carolyn wants Momma well, but not too well.

In reality Carolyn is scared. She has been subjected to many lies and empty promises from her mother. The idea of Shirley getting off disability is especially *scary since one of Shirley's roles is to bring that disability money into the house. In short, Shirley's job is to stay disabled!*

Obviously, there is more to this story, but the point here is that secondary gain can be received by the identified patient as well as those within the family system.

Addiction is a family disease. Chronic pain is a family disease.

Treatment of Chronic Pain: If you have chronic pain and are addicted, non-narcotic treatment of chronic pain is an important part of your recovery process. As an addictionologist, I do consult with other physicians who are pain specialists. They have non-narcotic interventions and procedures that can offer relief.

Medication management of chronic pain should target the mechanism of the chronic pain rather than just covering the pain up or making you less aware of it with opiates.

Realistic goals are important. The goal is to dampen or control the pain. If any healthcare provider tells you all your pain is going away, RUN!

Some of the medications that can be beneficial include:
- Duloxetine (Cymbalta)
- Pregabalin (Lyrica)
- Gabapentin (Neurontin)
- Non Steroidal Anti-inflammatory Drugs (NSAIDS)
- Baclofen
- Flexeril
- Elavil
- Vitamin D in large doses

- Topical preparations and patches
- Other antidepressants
- Antibiotics (yes, long-term antibiotics for chronic pain)

This is not an all-inclusive list. These are some of the medications I prescribe for chronic pain. There are other medications that can have beneficial effects on chronic pain.

If you have a co-existing diagnosis of addiction and chronic pain, you may notice that the more time you have away from the opiates, the less severe your pain becomes.

Other treatment considerations for chronic pain include:
- Training in relaxation techniques and physical rehabilitation (exercise). A common problem in chronic pain is the risk of deconditioning of muscles, bones, and joints
- Cognitive Behavioral Therapy – addressing maladaptive thinking (For example, identifying one's self as a "pain patient" may set up a self-fulfilling prophecy of being a victim. Self-talk is extremely important.)
- Understanding and dealing with the Fear Avoidance Model (FAM)
- Not smoking cigarettes or any other substance
- Meditation, guided imagery
- Biofeedback
- Massage therapy
- Transdermal Electrical Nerve Stimulation (TENS) units (now available over the counter)
- Acupuncture (equivocal in my eyes)
- Dealing with grief due the loss associated with chronic pain
- Remembering recovery takes time and is an ongoing process not an event

RATING RECOVERY

We have defined recovery and we have discussed various treatment components and options. The downward spiral into the abyss of addiction is not linear; therefore, it is not surprising that the recovery process is not linear either. Indeed, lapses and/or relapses are common, albeit not inevitable, characteristics of addictions.

Only about fifty percent of the people who enter a treatment program complete it. Some of these people will come back or get into another recovery process. Some will not. Some may recover without any intervention. Some may die. Some may end up incarcerated. Some may end up debilitated.

Whether you enter a self-help group, an outpatient program, a short term residential program, or a long term residential program, the results depend primarily upon your level of motivation to change. To that end, we will review two models for gauging the level of recovery and the prognosis for same.

For many years, addiction therapists relied upon the Grief Model to assess where the patient was in recovery and encouraged the patient to use it also. The Motivational Stage Model, put forth by Prochaska, et. al., has essentially replaced the Grief Model as a gauge for prognosis.

I present them both, because during your journey into sobriety, you will probably be introduced to both and they are not mutually exclusive. Use whatever works for you.

The Grief Model is based upon the fact that your primary "love object" has become your drug of choice. As such, when you successfully give up that love object, you will experience loss and go through a grief process.

Denial: the first level of grief. You do not believe there is a problem or that the problem is your relationship with a mood-altering substance. Therefore, you see no need to give up your love object.

> *"I need my Lortab, Xanax, Adderall, and Ambien, and I may have a glass of wine at night. But, there is no problem here."*

Bargaining: the second stage. It's also called the "Let's make a deal" stage. In bargaining you agree to sort of give it up.

> *"I will only drink beer." or "I am off the heroin and sticking to marijuana." or "I agree to stop drinking but I am still going to the casinos."*

Compliance: is the stage in which you agree to do something about "the problem."

Passive compliance occurs when you go to a program and just sit there as a spectator. This is not uncommon in people "court referred" to treatment.

With hostile compliance you are angry about not using, and you generally let everyone know about it. You may hear this referred to as "dry drunking." Hostile compliance is associated with statements like:

> *"I gave up drinking for you. What the hell more do you want?"*

Acceptance: is when you figure out you have a problem. Sometimes it is like someone finally turned on the light in your head.

> *"Hey, this is about me!"*

Surrender: is a word that turns many people off. The

interpretation of the word here is that you are no longer fighting yourself. You realize you have a disease and that you can recover and you do whatever is necessary to recover.

> *"I finally truly understand that I am allergic to alcohol just like I am allergic to penicillin. It would be stupid of me to get mad at the doctor if he refused to give me penicillin because we both know it would kill me on the spot. Penicillin would take me away from my family forever. So why would I not understand that people who care about me want me to avoid penicillin and alcohol. It's the same thing except I really never liked penicillin. But I really do get it now. Alcohol will take me away from them and hurt them and me. Fighting myself is not only futile and destructive, it is also stupid. What I really do not understand is how I could not see that before. This disease is a bitch!"*
> Marvin, 47 years old, husband, father of three children, and from down the bayou.

Another useful paradigm is the **Motivation for Change Model** which certainly has clinical utility. Here are the stages of change:

Precontemplation: This stage generally equates to denial in grief model. The person is unaware of any need to change his or her behavior. *"I do not have an addiction problem."* Generally, as the addictive process progresses, the consequences accumulate to the point that the person may enter into the next stage, but people can get stuck in this precontemplation stage and never move forward.

Contemplation: The person in this phase of change is beginning to wonder if there might just be a problem with his or her behavior. He or she may even try to alter the behavior somewhat. *"I will limit myself to 2 drinks and will only drink after 5 p.m."*

Preparation: The person perceives there is a problem, and treatment options are explored. That does not mean any treatment options are going to be chosen or utilized. This can also be a time for procrastination. The person may even bounce the idea of treatment off people close to him or her, like family members.

Action: The person chooses a recovery option and enters treatment.

Maintenance: In this stage, the person has achieved the desired behavior, such as sobriety, and now must work diligently to maintain this state.

Recurrence: not a stage per se but a return to the addictive behavior as in **relapse**. By definition, when there is recurrence, the person has moved out of maintenance and into one of the other stages but not necessarily back to the first stage.

These stages are not as straightforward as they might seem at first glance. A person can bounce back and forth between them. Hopefully, each bounce is a learning experience to prevent more bounces.

> Carl is a fifth-a-day guy. Being a cunning alcoholic, he only drinks vodka to disguise the odor of alcohol on his breath. Carl thinks vodka makes his alcoholism invisible. (You know the type. You may even be the type.) His liver enzymes are up and his relationships with his wife, children, and employer are down. He is coming off of a seven-day detox and heard

about some anti-craving medication in group.

Carl is 53 years old and has this to say about life: *"It is too late to start over. I have got to stop drinking. All I am doing is hurting myself and everybody else."* Not only has Carl lost a lot, he realizes that he is on the verge of losing everything else important to him. So he tells me, *"I want to do whatever it takes to stop."*

Judging from this presentation, it would be appropriate to place Carl in the Action phase of recovery. He accepts the fact that he has the disease of alcoholism. He sees the past, harmful consequences of his drinking and realizes those to come if he continues to drink. He came in only "to detox," but he is now seeking additional treatment. Let us delve a little deeper into his commitment to action.

I respond, *"That's great, Carl. The medication you are referring to is Antabuse. There are some possible side effects we need to chat about such as drowsiness, metallic taste in your mouth, rare decrease in sexual ability in males…"*

Carl bolts upright in this chair. *"Whoa up right there, Doc. You can forget me taking that stuff. I have got to be able to have sex with my wife."*

I respond that the sex side effects are rare, but Carl has selective hearing. He is adamant that a prescription for Antabuse is off the table.

Since it is such an issue, I have to ask the question. *"Carl, when was the last time you were sexually intimate with your wife or anyone else for that matter?*

"It was the last time I sobered up. Let me see.

Hmmm. Maybe a year or so ago." He pauses and shrugs his shoulders. *"I cannot remember, but I tell you what, if I cannot stay sober, I will come back and get some of that stuff from you, I promise."*

Where would you put his stage of motivation now? He is willing to do some things, but he is not willing to go to any lengths to get sober. Some would say he has already planned his relapse because he now sees Antabuse as a bargaining chip when he relapses. Some would say he is "trying to run his own program." After all, the addicted brain is very cunning.

I think Carl is vacillating between contemplation and action at this point, and I see him as more on the action side.

His wife would disagree and she wants him on Antabuse. And yes, her motives are multifactorial.

If Carl gets into a maintenance phase and practices recovery behaviors and strengthens recovery circuits and dampens addiction circuits, he will come to accept his sober behaviors as the norm, as will his family and friends. While each minute of recovery increases your chances for sustained sobriety, a milestone of five years is associated with a greater chance of lifelong sobriety. I say this because many professional boards require five years of monitoring, and their recovery percentages after that process is right at ninety percent in the success column.

Carl's recovery program illustrates that these recovery stages (both motivational and grief) are not sharply delineated. Change, recovery, transition or whatever other label you might use is a process, and it is often a vacillating one. When a loved one, an employer, a judge, or the patient asks me about the level of a person's recovery, I cannot give an exact measurement. What I can do is assess the commitment to change, as well as the person's biological, psychological, social, and spiritual asserts. The stronger the assets are, the more probable the strength and longevity of recovery.

The recovering person must be actively involved in this appraisal and monitoring because recovery is a dynamic and ongoing process. He or she also needs feedback from reliable and caring persons. You need to know where you are in order to gauge your progress and reinforce what is working.

Here are some of the factors involved in assessing prognosis.

Biological factors to take into consideration are multiple and varied. A patient who is going to require major surgery and narcotic medications would be more a risk for craving and/or relapse than a person who will not be exposed to them. Brain damage due to drugs and/or injuries is another risk factor. Chronic pain is a risk factor. Liver disease including Hepatitis C is a risk factor. There are multiple risk factors from a physical perspective. The key is to establish a liaison with a knowledgeable healthcare professional and follow through with a treatment plan you have input into.

Social factors include home environment, marital status, employment status, employment skills, supportive relationships, involvement in a recovery community, and financial assets. For instance, if you are an alcoholic and a compulsive gambler, you probably should not get a job as dealer in a casino.

Psychological factors include any mood disorders such an anxiety disorder, bipolar disorder and/or depression. ADHD, personality disorders, and/or thought disorders are also predictive of staying sober and in a maintenance phase.

Spiritual factors include being in sync with your values and perception of a power greater than self. Many addicts initially struggle with differentiating the concepts of religiosity from spirituality.

This brain malady we call addiction can rob an addict of the ability to adhere to his or her own ingrained values. This lack of adherence to values results in performing various behaviors the person feels are innately wrong. These violations of a person's moral code, takes a heavy toll. In Alcoholics Anonymous it is often referred to as "spiritual bankruptcy."

Spirituality is a difficult term to define. It is so personalized that it may indeed defy definition. Spirituality is one of those things that you know when you have it and you also know when you have abandoned it. I believe our brains are "hard wired" to seek out meaning and to transcend to a plane that is higher than mere existence. In order to do that, we must have intact brain circuits. This in turn means that if a person is actively addicted, the drugs are tying up the very circuits needed to move toward spirituality. The result of this "spiritual disconnect" is to promote behaviors that violate personal values and subsequently promote moral decay. The addicted brain, as a defense of the addiction, will begin to devalue its own ingrained spiritual concepts and values. This can result in an ongoing internal conflict best described as a battle between spiritual or real self versus the addicted self. These addicts describe it best.

> *"It is like I have these voices in my head. But I know they are not real voices. One tells me what I am doing is wrong and the other tells me 'what the F***" go ahead and do it.' I know I am a better person that what my behavior shows. I come out of the drug fog every now and then and feel so guilty that I would rather use to escape the pain than face what I have become."*

"I have strayed so far from who I am, or was, that I do not think I can forgive myself. I cannot even ask God to forgive me."

"I get up every morning and tell myself I am going to do the right thing. I used to ask God to help me, but I kept screwing up so much that I decided it was two-faced of me to pray not to use when I knew I was going to go use. So now I just get up and tell myself I am nothing but crap if I use today. I guess I am nothing but crap."

"I had sobriety once. And I was spiritually connected. I desperately want that back again. But when I blew it, the drug became my god."

"God? I have no God! I have no soul! I used to believe in that crap, but all I have now is guilt and fear and shame. I use heroin because I am an addict, and the damn drug does not even work anymore. And that is why I tried to kill myself, Doctor. Do you not understand that I am empty and I have nothing? Which means I have nothing to live for."

Spirituality actually offers protection against addiction. We previously discussed the reasons adolescents use mood-altering substances in the first place, and one of the main reasons is acceptance of drug-using behavior by the adolescent's peers. Research has continued to support the fact that a religious foundation is protective against adolescent drug use. Adolescents who have a religious foundation, as a group, are less likely to participate in the risk-taking behaviors of using alcohol or drugs. Religious involvement decreases the risk of addiction.

Spirituality in treatment appears to maximize recovery outcome. As a matter of fact, in one study, the ability to connect spiritually and to forgive self and ask forgiveness from God and others was a strong predictor of a positive outcome to treatment. This certainly supports my own personal bias that a person involved in a 12-step program should complete Step 5 and then follow up immediately with steps 6 and 7 prior to moving into any sort of aftercare. Not only have I witnessed the change in a recovering addict after a good Step 5, 6, and 7, I have experienced it myself. The weight can be lifted and the spiritual connection made with that experience. With this experience comes hope and forgiveness.

One caveat is important. Just because the weight is lifted, does not mean the disease is over. Recovery is an ongoing process. Practice is required to solidify that spiritual connection. That is why AA has maintenance steps. Life has maintenance steps.

Spirituality appears to increase the development and functioning of the prefrontal cortex of the brain. You will remember that this is the part of the brain responsible for the executive functions such as decision-making. The improved efficiency of the prefrontal cortex results in less impulsivity, greater moral reasoning, and the increased ability to act within one's value system. This in turn leads to behaviors compatible with one's values which equates to less anxiety, less shame, less guilt, and more emotional stability. Interestingly, a strong connection may decrease activation of the pain circuits within the brain. These circuits have been tracked by functional magnetic resonance imaging (fMRI).

Spirituality improves treatment response in those who have depression and appears to protect against recurrence of depression. I suspect that spiritually enhances mediation effectiveness in such patients via brain circuitry and brain chemicals that impact emotions.

As stated earlier, I believe spirituality is a very personalized experience that must be defined within the individual. I believe this brain disease overtakes the addict biologically, psychologically, socially, and spiritually and that in order to reach optimal recovery, each area must be addressed. Use of addictive drugs induces false emotions. I once had a patient tell me that heroin made her feel like she was in a field of yellow daisies, but they were all plastic. She also said the yellow was *"fading like cheap plastic flowers do."* I submit to you that addictive drugs are not only producers of false emotions, they are also akin to very destructive false gods.

RELAPSE

Lapses and **relapses** are common occurrences in the early stages of any desired change. Some therapists do not make a distinction between the two. I do. When I first heard about "slips" in my early days of recovery, I was terrified. I had just come through treatment hell, and things were getting better, and I had some direction and hope for my life when seemingly out of nowhere, I overhear these guys talking about a thing called a "slip chip." My brain was still foggy, but I knew that if they had a chip for slips, it must occur with some regularity. It scared the hell out of me because hearing that made it very real to me that I could fall back into that ever-waiting black hole of addiction. I was confronted with the stark realization that treatment does not guarantee recovery. I also realized that I had to keep doing the "right things" with the tools I got in treatment to keep my recovery going and growing.

Lapse My definition of "lapse" is a transient return to the non-medical use of a mood-altering substance. It is usually triggered by exposure to some internal or external event that is referred to as a "using cue."

For instance, if John has three months of sobriety and decides to gobble down a couple of Xanax when he opens his mother's medicine chest, he just lapsed. It was an almost spontaneous response to a familiar cue.

> *"The Xanax was there, and the 'old me' just grabbed the bottle real fast and took two pills. It was like someone else had opened that medicine chest and taken those pills. I know that sounds nuts."*

What John does next will determine if this lapse will become a relapse.

Scenario Number One: If he views his ingestion of the pills as a slip and a signal to get back into recovery immediately, he might exhibit this behavior.

> *"I could not believe I did that. It was like an automatic response. I was not thinking. I did not play the whole tape through. I started shaking and tried to make myself throw up. No luck. I fumbled my phone out of my pocket and pressed the speed dial for my sponsor. I told him the truth. He told me he was coming over. He and I sat down with my family, and I told them what just happened, and I told them how sorry and scared I was. We decided I needed to go to ninety meetings in ninety days and check with my addictionologist and aftercare counselor. I am back on track now."*

Scenario Number Two: Now we will look at what might happen if John is programed to view a lapse as a total loss of recovery. First off, he will now consider himself to be in full-blown relapse. He could easily extend that line of self-defeatist thinking into going on a binge as part of a self-fulfilling prophecy.

> *"So I said to myself. Well, I just blew it. Then all the old thoughts came back:*
>
>> *I'm back to ground zero.*
>> *I'm a failure.*
>> *Everyone is going to be me mad at me.*
>> *My wife is leaving me for sure this time.*
>> *My mother will be so disappointed.*
>> *They are going to send me back to treatment.*
>> *What the hell? I may as well go for it (relapse)!*
>
> *Then, I took the bottle and put it in my pocket and got out of there. I stopped on the way home and*

*drank a couple of beers then got stopped by the cops
and now I'm in a world of hurt."*

I for one prefer the first scenario, and I am sure John and his family would agree. The expectation for John, and any other addict for that matter, is commitment to making progress in recovery not to being perfect.

Here is something else to consider. His family did not shame or punish him for coming forward and doing the right thing. They did not condone his behavior or blow it off as no big deal. They expressed appropriated concern and encouraged him to take his sponsor's advice; and they held him accountable. Had they shamed him, he would be less willing to be honest with them should something like this happen again. That might prompt him to go underground and to lie. That would prompt a relapse cycle. Please, don't misinterpret what I am saying. It is John's responsibility to stay sober, but it surely helps when family members are aware of the disease process and know how to respond accordingly and appropriately.

Relapse Triggers: There are people, places, and things that become associated with using alcohol and/or other drugs. Exposure to such cues can create cravings. These triggers can just come out of the blue sometimes, or so it seems. There are internal and external triggers. Internal triggers can be emotional and/or physical. For instance, if you have a bad headache, you might just remember how Lortab makes pain go away, especially if Lortab is your drug of dependence. Emotions may also serve as triggers.

There are seven basic or primary emotions that we all normally have. We spend most of our time in an emotional state of acceptance or neutrality. The other six primary emotions are happiness, surprise, disgust, anger, sadness, and fear/anxiety.

Men tend to relapse when experiencing positive stressors or emotions like happiness.

> *"Man, I am really feeling good. The game was great. Our team won. I got a raise yesterday. Life is good. I need to celebrate. I will just have a couple of beers. Yep. I will limit myself to just two!"*

Women, on the other hand, tend to relapse behind negative stressors and negative mood states.

> *"The house is upside down and I cannot get the kids to do a damn thing. My mother is calling 24/7 wanting me to babysit her blind 14-year-old Chihuahua for a week and I am PMS-ing. Screw it. I need a drink."*

Internal triggers can even happen in your sleep in the form of a "using dream."

A using dream is just that. You dream you are performing some part of your using ritual, either using or getting ready to do so. Sometimes these dreams wake you up abruptly.

> *"I woke up drenching wet with sweat and thinking I had used and blown my whole treatment! I was in a panic until I realized it was a dream."*

There are various interpretations of using dreams. They may be part of a grief process, or they may be related to fear of relapse; or they may just be a dream. I tell patients to not give them any power and to move on. I also ask them to talk very briefly about them and not get into romanticizing them. The reason I encourage talking about using dreams briefly is that I have found some people feel guilty about having one. Others hide the fact because they are afraid it might make others think they are insincere about recovery. A using dream does not mean you are going to use.

External triggers come in all forms shapes and sizes. For me it was a red ice chest and not just any red ice chest, mind you, but a specific brand and size. Every time I would see one, I would develop x-ray vision, and I could see right inside it. Inside everyone I saw was a case of iced beer. Yep. I could see the condensation on the can and feel the cold metal in my hand and taste that first icy gulp. This would happen to me wherever I came upon one whether it be on the shelf at a sporting goods store, at my kid's soccer game, or even in the back of someone else's pickup truck in a parking lot.

This experience would really make me mad at myself. I hated the power a random red ice chest had over me. How in the world could seeing a red ice chest make me want to have a beer and lose my family, wife, job, money, and self-respect? Here is how.

For years my father had a red ice chest and it was always full of beer. He took that thing everywhere. We drank together. When I was in the midst of my addiction, I followed suit and got my own red ice chest just like his, and that red ice chest became associated with getting hammered. Having a red ice chest was part of my using pattern or using ritual, so much so that when I was into early recovery and would see any red ice chest, two of my brain chemicals would activate.

Glutamate would be released and cause me to get excited. A very small amount of dopamine would also be released into my reward system and give me a little rush of pleasure in anticipation of more and greater pleasure to come by boozing it up. That glutamate/dopamine automatic response did not just go away because the judge and I agreed that I needed to stop drinking and drugging. There is also the fact that during my using days, I had trained my brain that once I had primed my reward center pump, I was on a mission to get that ice chest opened and drink that beer, and nothing was going to stop me. Unfortunately, my friend Raymond found that out about me the hard way on a fishing trip one August.

Ray's job was to get the beer. How hard is that, right? Anyway, he assured me he had accomplished his assignment, and we were ready to go. We loaded the boat, put into the water, and set out for about a thirty-minute trip. We arrived at our destination and weighed anchor. I was ready for a cold one, so I popped the top of the ice chest, and what the hell did I see? I saw a pitiful little six-pack of twelve-ounce beers sitting on a mountain of ice. I went nuts. I yelled at Raymond and called him a cheapskate and other choice names that I wish I could retract. I was smoking with rage. My addicted brain told me that Raymond was blocking my alcohol euphoria and thereby threatening my very survival. Raymond thought we were out there to fish! That idiot! We both got angry and the trip was over, but not before I guzzled down those six beers on the way into the dock. I was not letting that jackass have any. It was a bad time. I drank about it for days.

Once I got into recovery, I had to go make amends to that man and let him know I was the idiot.

As time and sobriety went on, the sight of a red ice chest lost its power over me. I would see one and laugh (internally) about how crazy I had been. Now when I see one, I realize how grateful I am.

There are some external triggers that are overwhelming and need to be avoided. For instance, if you are an IV drug user and you share an apartment with three other people who are shooting heroin, your chances of staying sober are nil. Your sobriety can not afford to be around the drugs or the druggers.

You also do not need to be around marijuana addicts even if your drug of dependence is oxycodone, amphetamines, or alcohol. If you start with a toke, you may learn that addiction is not about a specific drug, a specific type of drug, the amount of a drug, or the frequency of use. Addiction is about the brain's reward circuitry. That is why the use of any mood-altering substance can reactivate your pathological addictive brain circuits and can lead you back to your drug of choice.

An addictive brain can certainly be baffling at times. I have actually treated patients who intentionally used to get back into treatment.

> "I only used once this time, I did not want to spin off into my addiction again. But, when I was here in treatment, I knew I needed to deal with that secret but I just could not bring it out. It is been eating at me even more since I do not have drugs to cover it. So, I decided to use so I could check back in here and deal with it this time."

Crab Addicts: This crab parable was told to me in 1978 shortly after I got out of residential treatment. What brought it on was that I was defending my right to hang with my old "drinking friends" at my favorite pub and drink nonalcoholic beverages.

I think my counselor told me this story because he knew I went to the beach occasionally and that I liked to wander along the shoreline and pick up crabs for dinner. It was actually a family thing. The point being is that he was a master at visualization techniques. It worked; hence, I'm sharing it with you 35 years later.

There are these two guys walking down the

beach at Gulf Shores. Each has a bucket. The plan is to pick up crabs and boil them for dinner. They have pretty good luck and pick up a bunch. As the sun sets, they head back. One of the guys notes that his bucket is only half full because half his crabs have crawled out to safety. He looks at his friend's bucket and it is full to the brim. None of those crabs have gotten out. Perplexed, he asks why none of his friend's crabs have crawled to safety and avoided the boiling fate that awaits. *"Simple,"* his friend says. *"I only pick up addict crabs. That way when one tries to crawl out, the others pull him back in."*

Point made! I never did go back into that bar, but I have helped a couple of those friends from there get into recovery. Recovery truly is a program of attraction.

Unfortunately combining that attraction with our own false pride, can be a real killer for us. Which brings us to another, deadly relapse "sin" called the "rescue fantasy" syndrome - when you decide to go out and save everyone else from their addiction(s). Learning recovery skills is similar to learning how to swim in that if you have not learned to swim well, you probably should not jump into the ocean to save someone who appears to be drowning.

"I had been out of treatment for two weeks when my sister asked me to go talk to her husband. He was a drunk. But, he did agree to meet me at the Hilton. He was staying there because she had kicked him out again. Of course, when I got there I found him in the bar. But, what the hell, I went in and sat on the stool next to him. The barroom itself was almost intoxicating. I did not realize how much I had

missed the sounds, the low lights, and the smells. I sat there with him while he guzzled down Jack with Diet Coke, and we started talking about alcoholism. After about twenty minutes, I realized I was on my sixth glass of Diet Coke, and I was getting into the ambiance of the place and getting thirsty! What the hell was I doing? I stood up, told brother-in-law that I was sorry, I have got to leave, and if he wants some help, to give me a call because I was out of there. I got into the car, called my sponsor, get a good chewing out about powerlessness, pride, insanity, and stupidity, and made a meeting that night. He told me about how there were ways to make a 12th step call, and what I had just done was not one of them. I had been in that environment for twenty minutes, and I was thinking about blowing everything I had worked so hard for. Oh yeah, about brother-in-law, he actually went to treatment a couple of weeks later and is still sober.

Miracles happen, but the biggest miracle is that I did not relapse. That was really stupid on my part. I had bad cravings for a month after that." As told by Ted, recovering alcoholic, 31 years old, six months into sobriety, sharing his story in aftercare

Sex and Relapse: It was considered sage advice when I was a newcomer not to make any major life-changing decisions if they could be avoided. I still consider that to be a solid premise. One major decision is entering into a new sexual relationship. Here are some of the reasons for not doing so.

Sex activates the same reward pathways as addictive drugs. That is not exactly a news flash, but it does give cause for concern. A newly recovering addict could easily fall into the trap of using sex as a drug substitute. Multiple partners and compulsive sexual behaviors lead to all sorts of complications and high-relapse risks.

This dangerous and dysfunctional behavior has been recognized in AA for years. It even has a discreditable name. It is called "step thirteen." This is not a real AA Step. There are only twelve steps. Step thirteen refers to the unacceptable behavior of seeking out sexual partners in AA. Such behaviors often end badly. Unfortunately, there are many vulnerable newcomers, and there are predators who prey upon them. There are also people there with co-existing personality disorders who tend to act out their personality disorder behaviors, especially the Clusters B and C we talked about.

Most recovering people can understand that what we just talked about is true for "just sex" but what about true romance? If your coping mechanism and primary love object has been a drug, you are in no way ready for a new romance. The illusion of a treatment romance and/or a recovery romance can be fostered by the recovery atmosphere. People who are thrown together to combat the common disease of addiction (or any other) often find themselves in an open and sharing environment. They share secrets with others that they previously feared would yield only rejection. They are not rejected by the group so they bond to those members. Sometimes that bonding can be misinterpreted. This is one reason I prefer gender-specific groups.

If you get into a treatment romance, the fantasy world takes over, and you defocus from your own recovery program. When the fantasy does not play out and the "romance" ends, the rebound is a major relapse trigger especially since your recovery skills were linked to that fantasy.

Relapse cycle: I have heard this relapse history so many times that I feel a need to share it because it may provide you with insight on how to avoiding relapse cycling.

> *"I am not really sure why I relapsed. I know I got bored with all the recovery stuff. Then I got complacent and stopped doing all the things that were keeping me off drugs. You know, like going to meetings and calling my sponsor and hanging out with people in recovery. I got with some old friends and had a beer, and it went okay. So I did it again a couple of times without any problem. Then I got back into the whole addiction. Now I am back here in detox."*

It is not uncommon for me to hear the word boredom linked to relapse. As a matter of fact, I was whining about boredom one time early in my recovery, and my sponsor took it upon himself to define the word "boredom" for me.

> *"Boredom is the feeling that the entire universe exists to entertain me, the center of the universe. It is a reflection of total self-centeredness and self-pity."*

My sponsor was not exactly a subtle guy. He also told me to do service work and to stop being a spectator in recovery. That way, he said, I would not have time to feel bored, and maybe I could feel grateful. He was right. Then again so was that red neck preacher I heard at a tent revival my grandma dragged me to up in North Louisiana. He said that idleness is the devil's workshop. Even as a kid that made sense to me and it still does.

Written Relapse Prevention Plan: We mentioned this earlier, but I believe this is critical enough to rate expanding upon it. Every addict needs a Written Relapse Prevention Plan. I would prefer to call it a Recovery Maintenance Plan. A relapse prevention plan (or Recovery Maintenance Plan) lets you apply what you have learned from your mistakes and hopefully from the mistakes of others. I consider it to be somewhat of a safety net to keep you from "twisting off" into active addiction.

You know what your high-risk situations are. They could be family reunions, holidays, high school reunions, anniversaries of bad events, anniversaries of good events, the deer camp, the company party, weddings, or a myriad of things. If you sit down and figure some of these out, you can have a game plan on how to stay sober if placed into a high-relapse-risk environment.

Brenda gets a knot in her throat as she reads the invitation to Aunt Sissy's 80th birthday party. A worried frown crosses her brow as she reads the hand written note from her cousin at the bottom of the card: *"We Have a New Margarita Machine."* Aunt Sissy raised Brenda when her mother died. Brenda's cousins are heavy drinkers, and every family event is "party time." Brenda would normally join them, but she has been going to recovery meetings for the last six weeks and now she has a dilemma.

She calls her sponsor whose first question *is "Do you have to go?"*

"Yes, I do have to go. She might not make another birthday, and I owe her. I love that woman, and I could never forgive myself if I did not go. I am going."

Her sponsor advises Brenda to *"get a plan"* and to process it with her and the group prior to the event. She does so and here is what happens.

Brenda arrives with her fiancé about thirty

minutes early. They park the car almost a block away, so they will not get blocked in. Brenda seeks out Aunt Sissy and visits with her. She also tells Aunt Sissy that she will have to leave early. Brenda plans to mingle a little, but she and her fiancé have arranged a "code" that she will use if she gets uncomfortable. She gets a non-alcohol drink to hold like a shield in order to ward off those cousins who will be offering her a drink.

After another thirty minutes she and her fiancé leave and have a nice dinner to celebrate her success. Brenda checks in with her sponsor as planned, processes the event, and they agree to go to a meeting the next day.

Brenda got through the initial part of the high-risk situation, but now she needs to process the event in order to guard against a post-event relapse. Going into that environment can have some delayed triggers. For instance, wandering though the party could trigger cravings and euphoric recall. Success can make you over-confident. Being around family members can trigger feelings of resentment, guilt, and/or shame which in turn can trigger cravings and relapse.

The written plan also needs to include what to do if you need to take mood-altering chemicals (remember Karen). Any mood-altering drug has the potential to trigger you back into your active addiction. The operative word in that statement is "potential." Just because you have to take a narcotic for a broken bone, does not mean you will reactivate your addiction; it simply means there is the potential to do so. However, if you end up in the Emergency Department with a broken femur, and the doctor has just ordered IV Dilaudid that is not the time to try and figure out a plan.

Your Written Relapse Prevention Plan should have an updated list of names and contact numbers of people who will help you.

> Who will dispense any mood-altering substances to you?
> Who will make sure your MD knows that you are in recovery?
> Who will contact your sponsor?
> Who will notify your addictionologist?
> Who will pick the kids up?
> Who will notify your employer if you are out a few days?

To assure your best chance for sobriety, it is a good idea to have some sort of contingency contract built in. Accountability breeds caution and recovery. A contingency contract can be as simple as, "If I relapse, I agree to go into detox immediately and get into a relapse prevention program."

Some contracts outline the amount of time a person will attend aftercare and the number of meetings he or she will attend. There should definitely be a drug-screening agreement of some type built into the plan.

One of the reasons for the high recovery rates achieved by doctors, nurses, pharmacists, and other healthcare professionals is accountability. They all have strict "recovery contracts" and adherence to those contracts results in a recovery rate of ninety percent five years after treatment. After five years of maintenance, the odds of staying that way are very, very favorable.

SELF-HELP GROUPS

We have touched on self-help groups prior to this section. My purpose here is to present a specific section that can serve as a reference guide (of sorts).

Alcoholics Anonymous, AA, started it all, and AA is the quintessential twelve-step mutual aid, self-help support group. I included things in this segment for the person who may be just starting out in AA and also for family members, so they can understand a little about AA. Some of you may already go to AA. Others may have tried it for a while and "matured out of it." Some go one or two times and decide it is not for them. Some stay with it for life. As with any organization of this sort, there are AA zealots at one end of the spectrum, and at the other end there are AA detractors who vehemently denounce AA as a cult. There are those who not only criticize the message but also criticize any messengers.

Resistance to AA participation often presents in the form of critical comments or opinions. The one I hear most often is that AA is a religion or even a cult. Some people are repelled by the "Higher Power" or "God" thing. It is almost as if they are saying AA has failed them by not conforming to their expectations. The twelve-step principles work for many people, and there are numerous non-AA adaptions of these steps. There is even a non-AA twelve-step adaptation for atheists, and the Big Book of AA has a chapter written for agnostics.

I have little or no tolerance for all this controversy. If AA works for you, do it. If it does not fit your needs, do not do it. AA will always be there if you decide to reconsider and give it another try. You can even go after you have criticized it. Much of the addiction recovery literature supports AA as a valuable asset to recovery, and those who get into it have a better chance at sobriety. Maybe people who get into AA recovery are a preselect group. Whatever. I suggest keeping an open mind and giving it a chance. After all, what is the down side? You can try it and never go back, or you and try it and go back. My sponsor told me to look for similarities and not differences in AA. He was right, and that worked for me.

There are all sorts of meeting options. There are gender specific meetings, young people meetings, Big Book study meetings, speaker meetings, open meetings, etc. AA is not an exclusive club, and family members may want to attend an open meeting just to check it out. With all the options and nuances, the newcomer needs some sort of guide. That guide is called a sponsor.

Most people start out with a temporary sponsor who may or may not become a permanent sponsor. It is a good idea to pick a sponsor with at least three years sobriety. Pick someone you are not sexually attracted toward. Ask the potential sponsor about other "sponsees" and talk to them. If your sponsor is not a fit, it is okay to change, and if your sponsor finds you are not a fit, it is okay for him or her to recommend you find a different sponsor. If your sponsor relapses, you definitely need a new one. If your sponsor does relapse, do not personalize it. You are going to have a lot of contact hours with this person – daily phone calls, one-to-one meetings to work the steps, attendance at a home group. Speaking of a "home group", this is the meeting you chose as sort of an AA base. You will be expected to perform "service work" such as setting up chairs and the like at first. Like the slogan says: "You can't keep it unless you give it away." That is one of the reasons sponsors do what they do.

If you have been in a formalized treatment program, you may have been told to go to ninety meetings in ninety days. If not, your sponsor may have you do the ninety in ninety.

I do not know many people who just got up one day and walked into AA alone, especially if they have social anxiety. The first time out, most people go to a meeting with someone they know. Obviously, that someone is usually involved in recovery.

Some people get introduced to AA while in a treatment program. AA is not treatment per se. AA is not about giving advice, it is about sharing. If AA is a fit, you will find it to be a safe haven in which you, the recovering addict, can be accepted, understood, and not judged. If you participate, you will not only help yourself, you will also help others and allow others to help you.

You do not really "join up" in that you do not sign in, but you are welcome to join in. AA is free and it is anonymous, at least that is one of the principles. Anonymity is relative. People are human. Have realistic expectations. While it is supposed to be a voluntary experience, in reality people do get pushed into AA. Attendance may be court-ordered or mandated by some recovery contracts via licensing boards. Attendance may also be a requirement for being in a treatment program or for living in a "sober house."

The basic message, philosophy, and format of AA are universal. However, different meetings tend to take on individual characteristics. There are meeting guidelines, but each meeting has a degree of autonomy. It's like an evolutionary process. If the AA meeting is in an older, stabilized community, the members may be older and more stabilized than a 19 year old who shows up with a Mohawk haircut, a baseball cap on sideways, and half pound of metal in his face. That 19 year old probably will not fit well into that meeting, but if he is serious about recovery, he won't get kicked out either. You need to shop around to find the right type of meeting.

AA is not perfect. Nothing is. It is what you make of it. If you are trying to get into recovery, get an Alcoholics Anonymous "Big Book," read it and see if it fits. The book is not very expensive. It is cheaper than a six pack.

Narcotics Anonymous is the counterpart to Alcoholics Anonymous. As previously noted, there was a time when some AA groups did not allow you to mention your drug addiction, but you could talk about your alcoholism. Narcotics Anonymous was, in part, a natural outgrowth of AA. Indeed, it was initially called AA/NA. There are over 60,000 NA meetings worldwide.

As a note, many people addicted to alcohol and other drugs go to AA and are readily accepted there and do well there. Like I said, you may have to shop around to find the right fit for you.

Al-Anon/Alateen meetings are also known as Al-Anon Family Groups. The purpose of these meetings is to help family members of alcoholics. The concept of family extends to include concerned or significant others of alcoholics. Al-Anon is for adults. Al-Anon sponsors Alateen groups for teenagers. These are twelve-step programs. From my experience, the majority of Al-Anon members are women. I do not find this surprising since women are more likely to seek help within a group environment. Women also tend to be more supportive of their addict partners. Al-Anon was actually founded by Anna B and Lois W. (Lois Wilson) who was married to Bill Wilson, one of the founders of AA. Supposedly, Bill W. encouraged Lois to launch Al-Anon. There is scientific research to show that participation in Al-Anon can improve the quality of life for some of its members.

Celebrate Recovery (CR) is a biblical/church-based

recovery program. It has been around for twenty odd years and is in over 20,000 Christian churches nationwide. I have talked to people who embrace CR and seem to have established a solid recovery within the CR structure. CR is not AA. AA is a spiritual program that encourages you to define your own High Power. The Higher Power in CR is Jesus Christ. If you are looking for a faith-based recovery process, Celebrate Recovery seems to be pretty sound. Like anything else, you may have to shop around for a CR group that is a fit for you.

Self-Management for Addiction Recovery or SMART is more "science based." I like the Cognitive Behavioral Approach SMART offers. My problem with SMART is that meeting availability is sparse albeit you can tap into SMART via internet. They offer some good literature. SMART can interface with AA, NA, and/or CR.

From what I have seen and experienced, no matter which one or more of these you chose, the basic principles hold true, and none of the above are exclusive of the others. I recommend patients who are addicted to alcohol and/or other drugs start with AA and go from there.

There are other "specialty" self-help groups available, such as Gambler's Anonymous, that I am not as personally familiar with either because I do not have that particular malady or because I do not treat those particular compulsions. However, I do know professional therapists who do treat them, and I can point you in the right direction.

SPECIAL HEALTH CONSIDERATIONS FOR ADDICTS

Hepatitis

Hepatitis is an inflammation of the liver. The toxic properties of alcohol can cause alcoholic hepatitis. Other toxins such as acetaminophen, various medications, plants, and industrial chemicals can cause a chemical hepatitis. Various virus infections can cause Hepatitis A, Hepatitis B, and/or Hepatitis C as well as Hepatitis D and/or Hepatitis E.

In my patient population, the most common method of getting Hepatitis C is through sharing contaminated needles and other contaminated IV injection equipment such as water, spoons, and/or filters.

The initial infection is called the acute phase. The signs and symptoms of the acute infection usually go unnoticed, especially if you are using dope and masking any symptoms. If you do have symptoms, and only about twenty percent of newly infected people have them, you may feel fatigued, and you may have some abdominal pain especially in the upper right part of your abdomen. Many people describe it as having flu-like symptoms. You may notice your urine is really dark, and you may even notice your eyes turning yellow. However, most people do not get yellow, and most people do not even know they are infected.

It is often difficult, if not nearly impossible, to delineate an infection time line in a person with Hepatitis C.

> *"I never really felt sick. My urine never got really dark. I have been injecting for about 2½ years now. I shared needles sometimes, but we always rinsed them."*

Always rinsed them? That may be an overstatement of even wishful thinking. Let us take a look at that statement. You are jacked up and nodding out, but you are sure you used appropriate sterile technique. No way. Or worse yet, someone else drew the dope up and shot your arm vein full of it. You have no idea if the filter was shared, or if the spoon was free of the virus. In short, you may never know exactly when or where you got HCV infection.

If you inject the Hepatitis C Virus (HCV) into your blood stream, your body will develop antibodies to fight the HCV. If we test your blood for the HCV antibody, we will probably not detect it for at least four weeks after the infection, and in some people we might not be able to detect it for six months or more. This means you could have the HCV infection, and you would not know you are infected for six months, and you would not know at all unless you get a follow-up test. Therefore, if you are at high risk and possibly got exposed and your HCV antibody is negative, you need to check it again in six months.

There is another test that may show the HCV infection within about two weeks after you get infected. This is the HCV RNA test. If this test is positive, you have the HCV infection in your body.

If you are found to have the HCV, another test is ordered to see what type of virus you have. We know there are at least six different HCV types, called genotypes. Some genotypes respond better to current treatments than others.

Hepatitis C is a slow moving disease. The "natural course" of the infection without treatment is very germane to our discussion here simply because many people do not even know they have it. You might be surprised to learn that four million people in the United States have been infected by

HCV. Four million is an impersonal number, so we can try to put that number into a local perspective. If you are in a packed LSU stadium, at least 1400 people in there with you have a Hepatitis C infection going on. It also means that about 850 of them (sixty percent of those infected) got HCV from illicit IV drug use.

That is indeed a serious number, and this is a serious infection. More people die of HCV than HIV in the United States. HCV is the number one cause for needing a liver transplant in the USA and in Europe. Some research predicts the death rate from Hepatitis C will increase over the next twenty years due to liver failure and/or liver cancer. Since this is such a serious disease, you might be shocked to learn that many addicts do not get follow-up care! You certainly should be concerned.

> *"I know you told me I have Hep C, Doc, but I really never followed up. I sort of put it off because I was not ready to go through all that treatment stuff. Then, when I went back to heroin, I said to hell with it. I have tried to be careful. I do tell people I share drugs with that I have it. My girlfriend already has it so we can share without worrying about giving it to each other. I guess I need to do something about it this time."* Julian is a 26-year-old heroin addict coming back into detox for the third time.

Prognosis: If you have the infection, this is your prognosis (or your odds) for progressive liver damage if you do not get treatment.

Fifteen to twenty-five percent of people infected with HCV actually clear the virus. That means your immune system will wipe it out, and you will be free of the virus and non-contagious. Pretty great news for those that clear it. Women tend to clear the virus better than men. Infants also clear the virus in about twenty-five percent of the cases.

That also means that eighty-five to seventy-five percent of the people infected will develop a chronic HCV infection. Five to twenty-five percent of folks with chronic HCV infection develop cirrhosis of the liver over twenty-five to thirty years. Women tend to get less severe liver complications. Thirty percent of the people who get HCV cirrhosis will get liver failure and one to three percent will get liver cancer.

HCV can also infect your brain. Chronic HCV infection can cause brain dysfunction. Your ability to make appropriate decisions may be blunted. You may have memory problems. You may have poor attention capability. You may feel fatigued. You may have significant depression and/or anxiety. Indeed, about sixty percent of people infected with HCV are depressed.

Treatment: Much effort is going into developing medications to treat HCV. With current medications, we are seeing a high success rates for some HVC genotypes. There is also a great deal of research going into developing new medications for HCV.

The treatment lasts six to twelve months. Females tend to have a better response to HCV clearance. These medications may have significant physical and mental side effects. Not the least of which is the possibility of depression. The depression can be controlled with antidepressant medications and ongoing counseling.

While medications are available, you and your physicians may elect to simply monitor you initially. Using a "watchful waiting" approach depends on many individual factors. Those factors include, but are not limited to, the stage of your liver disease and your willingness and ability to adhere to a treatment regimen which, as we all know, equates to your ability to stay sober.

Morphine has been shown to enhance the growth of the Hepatitis C Virus. Obviously, using heroin or Roxicodone, or whatever opiate you like, makes things worse for you. Methadone and/or buprenorphine may not have this virus acceleration effect, but then again, we are talking about "therapeutic doses." If you are actively addicted, your life will certainly be unmanageable to the point that you will not adhere to the HCV treatment regimen, and you may end up with a mutated virus that becomes resistant to medications.

The last thing you need is to develop a resistant strain of the virus from poor medical compliance. Actually, that's the last thing the human race needs. Naltrexone injections may be worth considering if you have HCV and are getting medical treatment for it. Naltrexone may have some independent protective effect on a liver infected with HCV.

The important thing is that you establish a relationship with a physician and follow through with treatment and/or monitoring. Even if medications are not started right away, you will need to be vaccinated against Hepatitis A and Hepatitis B. You definitely do not want another liver virus infection on top of this one. Liver failure is a bad way to go.

Preventing HCV Infection: There is no Hepatitis C vaccination to date. Household contacts should avoid sharing razors or toothbrushes with HCV infected persons. What about sexual transmission? In heterosexual couples who do not stray from mutual fidelity, the rate of sexual transmission of HCV is one case per 190,000 sexual contacts.

Pregnancy and HCV: If mom is pregnant and has HCV infection, the risk of transmitting the HCV to her baby depends on the concentration of virus mom has in her body. Having a C-section does not appear to have any impact on whether or not the child will become HCV infected. The risk for passing the HCV from mother to child is about five percent.

Needles and Other Things

During my initial interview with an IV drug user, I always inquire about clean needles, dirty needles, shared needles, shared spoons, and shared filters. I also ask about the dope itself. What color was it? Did it dissolve easily? Was anyone else using the same batch? Did they get sick?

Needles and Syringes - Injectable use of opiates has been around since the invention of the medical syringe in 1854. While the syringes have changed, the addiction has not. Nowadays, heroin addicts usually use "insulin syringes." It is best to use a new syringe each time, but that is rarely the case for a variety of reasons. These syringes are relatively easy to acquire, but planning is not necessarily an addict's strongest personality trait either.

There is a lot of misinformation about syringes on the street. For instance, reusing the same syringe will not give the user Hepatitis C if he or she is the only person using it, but repeated use of the same syringe is going to cause some level of contamination of the syringe.

Human skin is an effective barrier against infections caused by viruses and bacteria. However, these germs are always present on our skins. That is why the nurse always scrubs your skin with an alcohol swab prior to giving you an injection. The scrubbing gets rid of the germs for short period of time. If this were not done, the needle might push some germs into your body. That could result in various types of infections including the formation of an abscess. If you are loaded up on dope, you are probably not using good injection techniques. That is one of the reasons addicts get infections.

Washing a syringe out with bleach offers some protection, but if you are sharing syringes, you are endangering yourself. If you do decide to bleach a syringe, make sure you flush all the bleach out of it before you use it. No amount of cleaning is going to make a used syringe a sterile syringe.

Another problem with reusing syringes is that the needle gets dull. If you look at the tip of such a needle under magnification, it looks like a jagged beat-up knife blade that reminds me of the edge of a carpenter's saw. This means that you are literally tearing through the skin and into the vein when you use it. This promotes more scar tissue and more potential for infection. Some of the needle re-sharpening techniques you might hear about on the street may actually make things worse because the sharpening material may get ground into the needle. When you use the needle, that stuff gets into you.

There are other injection dangers that an intravenous drug user (IVDU) needs to be aware of. Some of it relates to the contents of the drug itself. When I ask my patients about the contents of the powdered heroin they're using, the universal answer is "who knows?"

The Cut - Heroin is cut with just about anything, including but not limited to sugar, powdered milk, starch, or other drugs. In addition to "the cut" there may be other contaminants. Some street samples have historically been positive for cadmium which is a toxic metal that over time can cause bone and kidney damage. Evidently the cadmium contamination of heroin occurs during the manufacturing of heroin from the opium plant. There is not a whole lot of quality control in the jungle.

Some of the drugs used to cut heroin are really "out of the box" or out of the prescription bottle. There have been cases of heroin being cut with blood pressure medication. I guess anything in the medicine chest is okay when you need to cut dope. Unfortunately, that particular cut resulted in a flurry of emergency room visits due to toxicity. Years ago there was a contaminant that caused the IVDUs to develop a neurological disease called Parkinsonism. Fortunately, such "outbreaks" are few and far between, but it does happen.

Powdered heroin is never pure, but even if it was, it would still have germs such as bacteria, viruses, and even fungus in it. So many people in so many places have handled the stuff that it is impossible to know what is there. Heating it up in the spoon with water does not necessarily kill all of the germs.

Black tar heroin deserves special mention due to the risk of botulism contamination. Heating black tar heroin does not kill the botulism spores. Botulism causes progressive paralysis of the entire body.

The Filter - Powdered heroin is place in a spoon (or some other small metal container like a bottle cap) and a small amount of water is squirted on it. The water is seldom sterile. It is then mixed and heated. After that, the liquid is drawn up into the syringe through a piece of cotton or a cigarette filter. This solution is then injected through the skin and into a vein. Sharing filters or spoons is almost the same thing as sharing needles. Sharing any drugs or drug delivery devices is a good way to get hepatitis C or transmit it to someone else. The same holds true for HIV infection. Multiple users drawing up water from the same source can also increase their risks of infection.

Cotton Fever - A relatively sudden onset of fever usually within thirty minutes after injecting heroin is a characteristic of cotton fever. The victim generally has a rapid heart rate, difficulty breathing, headache, body aches, and feelings of panic.

"It was like I was going to die. A few minutes after

I shot up, I had this headache and chills. My whole body started jerking, and I felt like my heart was going to pound out of my chest. My boyfriend said my skin felt like it was on fire. I was really sick and scared. I waited a few hours and sort of slept it off."

Cotton fever is usually self-limiting which means it wears off or goes away on its own. It is not uncommon for my patients to report a history of past episodes of cotton fever. One of the things that will increase the risk of getting it is the practice of reusing cotton filters. The street reasoning for the filter reuse is to limit the loss of any heroin, however minuscule, that might be retained in the cotton fibers. Another problem is that in a moment of desperation, some addicts retrieve the trashed filters and try to "wash them down" to get some dope out of them. This is another bad decision. Not only will there be very, very, very little dope to be had, the risk of infection or of getting toxic is definitely heightened. Plus, the used cotton may actually break down somewhat, and then cotton fibers are drawn up into the syringe and injected into the bloodstream. These cotton fibers may have bacteria and viruses clinging to them and cause infections of the body including an infection on the valves of the heart called endocarditis. Unfortunately, knowing all this is not going stop a desperate addict from compulsive behaviors that place self in harm's way.

The most probable cause of cotton fever is the growth of bacteria on cotton fibers. The bacteria secrete a poisonous or toxic substance. It is the toxin that causes the fever. If symptoms of cotton fever persist for over a few hours, it could mean something else is going on like a generalized bacterial infection of the body.

As noted above, some of my patients have told me they just "shake it off and keep on using." One major problem with that course of action is that a condition called sepsis can have the same signs and symptoms as cotton fever, and you will not shake that off. Sepsis is an infection of the whole body that can have dire consequences including infections anywhere in the body – like an abscess in your brain.

Most addicts I treat tell me that they use cotton from Q-tips. As an aside, dental cotton is supposedly the safest. Then again, injecting heroin is not a safe practice.

Cigarette Filtering - Supposedly cigarette cotton filters are not as efficient as cotton. This type of cotton tends to break up easily, and fibers are pulled up into the syringe and subsequently injected into the bloodstream. These fibers carry germs and other particles and can get caught up in very small blood vessels and clog them.

I frequently see abscesses on the arms where an IV user "missed" and inadvertently injected around the vein or through the vein rather than into the vein. Usually these are "staph" bacterial infections. These infections may fill with pus and bacteria and therefore have to be incised (cut open) and drained of the pus. This procedure is called an "I and D" (incision and drainage). The incised wound is often packed with gauze-like drain to keep it open a day or two. The wound must be properly taken care of, and the drain removed when appropriate. The surgical procedure is followed by a course of antibiotics.

Overdoses - Heroin can shut down the center of the brain that tells us to breathe. Death by heroin overdose is usually due to respiratory arrest. The person simply stops breathing and essentially smothers to death. In the situation of a heroin overdose, providing mouth-to-mouth breathing can save that person's life. Unfortunately, the overdosed addict is usually not in the presence of people who know cardiopulmonary resuscitation (CPR). There are various "home remedies" on the street about how to treat a heroin overdose. The only effective way is to support the person's breathing and call EMS. There is an injectable medication called Narcan which can immediately reverse the respiratory arrest. There is also a nasally administered version. I am a proponent of needle exchange programs, but I have mixed feelings about handing out injectable Narcan to opiate addicts to have available in case one of their friends overdosed.

This idea is fraught with many problems including the fact that if an addict has a medication that he or she thinks can protect them from an overdose, he or she will be more likely to push the envelope and overdose.

> *"I get my buddy to stand right by me with the Narcan while I shoot up a super load of heroin just in case I might OD."*

Then again, I have some patients tell me they saved a friend who overdosed. I have patients who were saved by friends, and I have other patients who saw friends die of an overdose. However, I have also had patients who woke up next to a dead lover who overdosed. (Narcan would not have helped there.)

Like I said, I have mixed feelings about handing out Narcan to addicts, but I do not have the answer. It is a harm-reduction technique that can save a life, so at the end of the day, I come down on the side that it is probably better to make it available to narcotic addicts than to have them dying.

That entirely aside, heroin overdoses are acute medical emergencies. Respiratory assistance should be offered, but this should not delay calling EMS. EMS will subsequently administer Narcan and reverse the respiratory arrest. I agree that all first responders should carry Narcan.

Another problem with the respiratory depressing effects of heroin is the fact that a person can nod out repetitively to the point of developing a condition called anoxic brain damage. This simply means that there was a decrease supply of oxygen to the brain to the extent that brain cells died. The end result is of course brain damage.

Skin popping - The term given to injecting drugs such as heroin just under the outer layer of skin is called skin popping. Since the needle is not directly inserted into a vein, the initial surge of drug into the blood stream does not occur. Therefore, the brain is not flooded with the drug rapidly, and the rush is not as great. However, the effects of the drug may last a little longer with skin popping. This practice can result in getting all the same infections as with IV drug use. Abscesses are not uncommon with skin popping. Another medical problem is that scarring can occur just under the skin. This in turn decreases the blood and nutrients available to the skin and more skin damage and scarring can occur. This also means that if the user gets an abscess, it takes longer for the area to heal after the abscess is surgically drained. Physical examination of the injection area can reveal areas of discoloration and a generalized hardiness due to chronic scarring. Since skin popping results in chronic skin inflammation and infection, the user can develop a medical illness called amyloidosis which can result in severe kidney damage and ultimately end-stage renal failure. This means dialysis or a renal transplant will be needed to survive.

DRUG TESTING

Drug screening and testing should be a part of any ongoing recovery process. Drug testing alone is of little benefit unless the results are linked to consequences. Dirty urines should have negative consequences, and clean urines should have positive consequences. These consequences should be clearly defined up front, and all parties involved should be aware of them.

There are creative ways to fool a drug screen, and there are creative ways to detect that foolery. Since it is no secret among addicts on ways of beating a drug screen, I will present some of those tactics for the less informed people, like parents, who may be relying on drug screens to monitor compliance/abstinence.

Dilution is the most common method of defeating a drug screen. The idea here is that each drug screen has a certain cutoff level or concentration level in the urine. If the level is too low, the screen will not pick up on the presence of the drug and the test will be negative. If you drink enough water, your urine will become very diluted. If you dilute your urine enough, any recently ingested drug will be too diluted to meet the cutoff point concentration.

While that may sound like a good plan, it is not. We measure the urine concentration, and if it is too diluted, we consider the urine to be invalid. Some monitors consider a diluted urine to be a positive drug screen while other monitors consider two diluted specimens in a row to be a positive.

If you produce a diluted specimen, I could sit you out in the waiting room for a couple of hours without anything to drink. During that time, you will concentrate your urine to a level that will yield a valid specimen.

By the way, most of us in this business of drug screening, including me, have heard all the excuses for diluted urine.

> *"I drank a couple of bottles of water to be able to give a specimen. I just got off the treadmill and rehydrated. I take a diuretic (fluid pill) for my blood pressure. I'm a vegetarian."*

While an excuse may be valid, I will hold the person responsible for making sure they do not repeat the behaviors that cause dilution.

Many of the internet products sold to beat urine drug screens rely upon a diuretic effect.

Of course there is always urine **substitution**. You can sneak a urine specimen in with you, preferably a clean one. I know what you are probably thinking. Who would substitute a dirty urine with a dirty urine? You would be amazed. I have had substituted urines come back positive for drugs. Then the testee wanted a pass because it was not his or her urine to begin with. Good luck with that!

Some testing sites require a witnessed specimen. That means you have to urinate into a container while a monitor observes you. Males can buy a fake penis that connects to a battery powered hidden container of "clean urine." If they are not subjected to a protocol that detects such a device, they may indeed pass a witnessed urine collection. It is even easier for females. I know of one male physician who perfected the substitution method. He would fill his bladder with clean urine via a catheter and produce a clean witnessed specimen. His behavior was such that drug use was suspected and a hair sample obtained from him proved to be positive.

Then there is the **contamination** trick in which you put something into the specimen to change the test result. We check for contaminants.

Types of Panels and Tests: urine drug screens are not tests. A screen is not as specific as a drug test. Screens can have "false positives" from cross reactions with other substances. For instance, a urine drug screen may read positive for amphetamines when all the person took was an over-the-counter decongestant. If you perform a drug test on that same specimen, it will be negative for amphetamine. A drug test is specific and requires special testing machine, but for non-forensic drug detection, a screen is usually all that is needed.

Urine drug screens have limitations as to what will be detected. Make sure you know what drugs are included in the screening panel.

In a heavy user, marijuana may show up positive in a screen and a test for several weeks. There is a method to detect if the levels are falling as expected. It involves comparing urine creatinine levels with THC levels. If the levels do not fall as expected, it means the person is actively using marijuana.

By the way, if a person is not a regular marijuana user, the urine drug screen will only be positive for a few days if he or she uses the drug.

"Synthetic marijuana" or HMAs (herbal marijuana substitutes) is not detected with most urine drug screens. Synthetic marijuana can be screened for, but you must ask for a specific "test panel." Even then, the panel may not include the specific type of synthetic marijuana being used. Labs are getting better at this testing, but the synthetics change so frequently that it is a moving target.

Alcohol testing has made several relatively recent advances.

We can test the urine for two different compounds (EtG and/or EtS) to see if the person has been drinking within the past three or four days, we can also take a blood sample and test for a substance called PEth (phosphatidylehtanol) to see if the person has been binge drinking within the past two to three weeks.

Hair tests have pros and cons. An obvious "pro" is that contamination is difficult as is substitution. An additional "pro" is that hair can give a history of drug use over the past several months. One of the "cons" is that you have to have hair to test. I've had men show up at my office for an addiction evaluation who have shaved all their body hair off in anticipation of a hair drug test. The excuses for this get pretty creative also. Females may come in with white bleached hair or heavy dye jobs. Such presentations may prompt me to get a fingernail test or perhaps a polygraph.

Speaking of hair analysis, we can also check the hair of a newborn infant to see if mom used while pregnant.

There are more benefits to random drug screen monitoring than just trying to catch an addict using. For one thing, submitting to voluntary screening is a show of good faith on the part of the recovering person. It is also a safety net. If I know I may be drug tested tomorrow, I might be better prepared to resist a using trigger today. Accountability breeds caution and in this case success.

My younger participants have told me drug testing also serves to give them an honorable way not to use with peers. Of course, I do not want them around using peers in the first place. This is what one young man told one of his buddies who offered him marijuana, and it worked out well in his eyes

"Are you kidding man? You do whatever you want,

but my parents are drug testing me. If you think I am going to use, you are crazy."

Negative drug screens also create a track record of sobriety that can come in handy down the road. This is especially true if you happen to be a physician or a nurse or a recovering person involved in a custody battle. Of course, mandatory drug testing is part of the monitoring process for several years in the case of recovering healthcare professionals. This is definitely a contributing factor to a ninety percent success rate.

I will make one last comment on drug screening/testing. There are times when we do drug testing to make sure a person is taking a medication that is prescribed. For instance, prior to the availability of injectable naltrexone, we would monitor urine to make sure the person was taking the oral form as prescribed. Another use is to do a urinalysis on people taking Suboxone for maintenance just to make sure they are taking the medication and not selling it.

Drug screening and testing is not infallible. Every addict I have ever met can figure out how to get around it at times or for a while. However, to my knowledge none of those trying to cheat the drug test knew how to stay sober, and their behaviors ultimately betrayed the fact that they were using.

CLOSING REMARKS

When we defined "recovery", we talked about needing to manage one's disease. This brings up the notion of "chronic-disease management." In a nutshell this means availing yourself of community services, finding appropriate healthcare providers, enlisting support from others, helping others, and following the treatment plan you helped create.

I would like to pass on some wisdom imparted to me by my sponsor. He was a brilliant guy who had a dry sense of humor and twenty-something years of sobriety when I met him. The last time I saw him was in a hospital room a couple of days before he died of cancer.

I remember that I was about six months into my recovery when he asked me, *"What are you doing for fun?"*

I thought it was a trick question. Was this guy serious? I was working on recovery way too seriously to worry about having fun! Plus, I had no real answer. While I was searching for an answer, he threw another curve ball my way.

"You're turning into a workaholic."

Damn, just when I thought I was doing great. That hit me dead center because he was right. Like many addicts, my motto was "nothing in moderation" and that included work.

Sublimation is the process of converting a socially unacceptable behavior, like addiction, into an acceptable one, like work. Sublimation is also a "socially acceptable" trap for us. It can cause us to "get stuck." For instance, I can use my workaholism as a shield to deflect any criticism or concerns about my level of recovery. *"After all, look how hard I'm working for you all."* I can also use working too much to avoid having to deal with any issues that I'm uncomfortable with. I can also tell myself that I'm too busy to spend much time going to meetings.

My sponsor also said in a matter of fact manner, *"If you do not have fun, you will probably relapse, or you will end up being a dry drunk."*

My "fun times" had become enmeshed with drug use. I needed to learn or re-learn how to have fun without them, but I was actually at a loss. What's an addict to do? He wanted me to learn to have fun without drugs. Okay, I could buy that. He also wanted me to have fun in moderation. Wow! What is moderation? Does that mean I allocate fifty-five minutes for fun each day? I had no real concept of a balanced life because I relied on chemicals to balance me. We all know how well that worked out.

Here are some other words he left me with:

> *"When you think about using, and trust me, you will think about using, do not dwell on the how good it was. Play the whole tape thought to the bad part."*

> *"Using (relapse) thoughts only last a short time unless you entertain them. Don't!"*

> *"Listen to your fear. If you feel you are in a high-risk situation, you are. Get the hell out of there."*

> *"There are some people you need to stay away from. You know who they are."*

> *"Sometimes you just have to shake the dust off your feet."*

> *"I'm responsible TO you not FOR you."*

"If you cannot forgive yourself, you have no God."

"I am grateful my family got to know me sober and I got to know them sober, and I am grateful I am going to die sober."

GLOSSARY

(Why a glossary? Why not? That is how this one came to be.)

ACOA – Adult Child of Addict or Adult Child of Alcoholic.

Al-Anon – twelve-step, self-help support group for family members who have an alcoholic or addict in the family.

Alcoholics Anonymous – the original twelve-step, self-help recovery program developed in the 1930's and based on spiritual principles to help alcoholics recover.

Alcohol Contained in Cooked Foods - this is the alcohol burn off chart from the US Department of Agriculture:

alcohol added to boiling liquid & removed from heat	85%
alcohol flamed	75%
no heat, stored overnight	70%
baked, 25 minutes, alcohol not stirred into mixture	45%
Baked/simmered dishes with alcohol stirred into mixture:	
15 minutes cooking time	40%
30 minutes cooking time	35%
1 hour cooking time	25%
1.5 hours cooking time	20%
2 hours cooking time	10%
2.5 hours cooking time	5%

Anhedonia – the inability to experience pleasure in things that would normally produce enjoyment.

Big Book – refers to Alcoholics Anonymous book; the first book was big and it was red.

Blunt – cigar cut open and filled with marijuana

Catastrophizing – predicting bad things are going to happen and that there will be major damage.

Chips – small medallions used to mark recovery time. There is a "desire chip" for those just starting and a month chip, etc.

COA – Child of Addict or Child of Alcoholic.

Cognitive – relating to the process of thinking.

Concerned Other – refers to someone who cares about the addict, this may or may not include family members.

Dry Drunk – This non-scientific term refers to someone who is not using but still exhibits all the negative behaviors of being actively addicted. This often refers to someone who is angry about not being able to drink or use drugs. When confronted on such behaviors the standard answer is: "I'm not drinking, what else do you want from me?"

Emphathogen – a substance that induces strong feelings of empathy and connectedness.

Entheogenic – refers to drugs used in spiritual rituals or to achieve otherworldliness or to transcend the moral plane.

Fetus – Latin word for offspring or bringing forth or hatching of young

FOO – Family of Origin.

Friend of Bill W – An addict or an alcoholic. If you happen to be on a cruise ship and look at the list of events, you may see an AA meeting listed in the guise of a Friends of Bill W's meeting - I did. It was a pretty good meeting.

Harm Reduction - Harm reduction refers to measure used to decrease the consequences of IVDU. Such measures include needle exchange programs, Narcan distribution programs, methadone maintenance programs, and buprenorphine maintenance programs.

HIPAA - Health Insurance Portability and Accountability Act is the law that sets the standards for our right to medical privacy.

Home Group - primary AA meeting which an addict attends and does service work and helps maintain the meeting.

In his/her cups - from 17th century meaning "to be drunk."

Jail House Tattoo - **refers** to a "homemade" tattoo one got in jail. Workmanship aside, this is a good way to get viral hepatitis.

Learned Helplessness - the state of being conditioned to feel and act helplessly in a destructive situation even when there is opportunity to escape the situation; people suffering from learned helplessness just give up and assume a victim role.

Let go and Let God - short version of The Serenity Prayer (I say it a lot!)

Narcotics Anonymous - twelve-step, self-help recovery program for drug addicts, modeled on Alcoholics Anonymous.

On the pipe – Smoking crack cocaine or methamphetamine with a pipe usually made of glass.

One day at a time – AA slogan refers to "staying in the day and staying sober one day at a time." For some it is "one minute at a time." It is the opposite of "future tripping."

PETH phosphatidylethanol – blood test for alcohol consumption which can stay positive for up to three weeks after the last drink.

Pigeon – a newcomer in AA or a sponsee.

Pink Cloud – slang term for unrealistically thinking everything is wonderful and then crashing when the real world comes back into play.

Rig – equipment (syringe and spoon) to use drugs intravenously.

Robotripping – the act of drinking large amounts of Robotussin DM with the intent of experiencing stimulation, euphoria, depersonalization, distortions and/or hallucinations.

Roxies – Roxicodone/ oxycodone pills.

Scheduled Drugs –
- Schedule I – no accepted medical use and high potential for abuse such as heroin, LSD, MDMA
- Schedule II – medical drugs with high potential for abuse such as oxycodone, Adderall, Cocaine
- Schedule III – medical drugs with moderate potential for abuse such as hydrocodone, testosterone
- Schedule IV – medical drugs low potential for abuse such as Xanax (really!)
- Schedule V – medical drugs less potential for abuse

such as Lomotil
- <u>Drug of Interest</u> – medical drug not controlled but being tracked such as Tramadol

<u>Serenity Prayer</u> – "God grant me the serenity to accept the things I cannot change, courage to change the things I can, and the wisdom to know the difference."

<u>Significant Other</u> – an intimate partner.

<u>SMART</u> – Self-Management And Recovery Training is a self-help movement that relies heavily of cognitive behavioral therapy.

<u>Sponsee</u> – someone being mentored by another recovering person in AA who preferably has several years of sobriety and works a solid program.

<u>Sponsor</u> – person in a twelve-step program who will mentor another member; there are criteria for being and choosing such a person.

<u>Stinking thinking</u> – entertaining negative thoughts such as using drugs.

<u>Thirteenth Stepper</u> – an AA sexual predator.

<u>Traumatic Bonding</u> – a strong bonding that develops between two persons when one intermittently abuses the other; often seen in ongoing domestic violence situations.

<u>Twelve and Twelve</u> – refers to AA book "Twelve Steps and Twelve Traditions."

<u>Two Stepper</u> – an AA member who "works" only step one and step twelve; the short version is "I'm an alcoholic and I can tell you how to run your life." Avoid these people.

Made in the USA
Lexington, KY
28 December 2016